Occupational Therapy in Epidermolysis Bullosa

Hedwig Weiß

Florian Prinz

Occupational Therapy in Epidermolysis Bullosa

A Holistic Concept for Intervention from Infancy to Adult

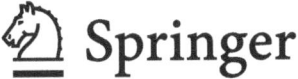 Springer

Hedwig Weiß MPhil.
Florian Prinz
University Clinic for Physical Medicine and Rehabilitation,
State Hospital Salzburg, Salzburg, Austria

SpringerWienNewYork is part of
Springer Science + Business Media
springer. at

Typesetting: le-tex publishing services GmbH, 04229 Leipzig, Germany

Printed on acid-free and chlorine-free bleached paper
SPIN: 80035976

With 154 (partly coloured) Figures

Library of Congress Control Number: 2012940859

Additional material to this book can be downloaded from http://extras.springer.com

ISBN 978-3-7091-1138-3 SpringerWienNewYork

Foreword

This book can be seen as a milestone in improving the communication between therapists, carers and clients with epidermolysis bullosa, because it describes the practical possibilities of occupational therapy and other physical and medical techniques and applications for children with the condition in a clear manner. This practical textbook is also easy for clients to understand so that it will motivate them to use it to check up on the measures and exercises they have learnt. In this way it presents a contribution to quality improvement and therapeutic efficacy.

Much gratitude is due to the authors of this elaborately crafted book for their tremendous commitment. On the one hand, they have been successful in analysing the experience they have gathered in 10 years of contact with clients and filtering out those successful measures and integrating them into an effective, modern and innovative therapeutic concept. On the other hand, through intensive interdisciplinary work they have made fresh discoveries which assist therapists to enable the better wellbeing of clients with this very, very irksome condition.

This experience can be passed on to the therapists of the clients as well as to their families through this book so that, on the whole, the time spent on intervention and care can be better used. With this condition, this also means a contribution towards minimising the sensory and motor deficits. As a member of the executive board of the University Clinic for Physical Medicine and Rehabilitation at the State Hospital in Salzburg, it is very important for me, on behalf of my colleagues, to express our sincere thanks and recognition to the authors for their achievement. Along with their enthusiasm and participation they have given countless hours of their evenings and free time to work on this ambitious project. Without this involvement the goal could never have been achieved.

The achievement of my colleagues fills me with enormous pride and I wish this publication, the product of their efforts, every success, and may clients with epidermolysis bullosa profit from it.

Prof. Dr. Dr. Anton Wicker
Director of the University Clinic for Physical Medicine and Rehabilitation at the State Hospital in Salzburg

Preface

It is a truly heroic challenge to present such a complex condition as epidermolysis bullosa in an understandable textbook, and it deserves compliment and recognition of the great effort, endurance and creativity.

When I was invited to participate in an interdisciplinary epidermolysis bullosa team as a representative of the University Clinic for Physical Medicine and Rehabilitation at the State Hospital in Salzburg, I just did not imagine that becoming so involved with this subject would lead to such an expansion. This was because most of our therapeutic work is in direct contact with the skin. How could this be possible with skin as delicate as a butterfly's wing? Now experience shows a range of unexpected possibilities. We dared to attempt different approaches, some of which have been replaced with better ones, to widen our possibilities of intervention with epidermolysis bullosa. That this work aroused great interest, incorporated new ideas and that there was hardly any literature on the subject surprised me very much. From the start it was clear to me that delays in both motor and sensory development must be considered and as far as possible avoided. On the one hand, the blistering of the skin averts unrestrained grasp in the full meaning of the word, and on the other hand, painful attempts deter the desire to explore. And so the affected child lacks experience. This has an effect on the natural motor development, which then exhibits deficits. The influence of the parents and carers plays a large role in this context. Often there is an overprotection which limits the freedom of action even more. All of these considerations have been incorporated into this book. Therefore, it only remains for me to express the hope that all those reading and using it will find the assistance and guidance they are looking for.

Dr. Margret Burger-Rafael
Assistant Medical Director and Head of the EB Team of the University Clinic for Physical Medicine and Rehabilitation at the State Hospital in Salzburg

Introduction

Working as occupational therapists in the University Clinic for Physical Medicine and Rehabilitation at the State Hospital in Salzburg, we are concerned with the treatment of children and youths with epidermolysis bullosa (EB). In close cooperation with EB House Austria (*EB-Haus Austria*), we have been able to widen our knowledge and practice step by step. Building on this experience, with time, we had the idea of writing it down for other occupational therapists, as there would appear to be no literature on the subject of occupational therapy (OT) intervention and management of EB.

We hope that, in the sense of a holistic OT approach, this book offers possibilities for a comprehensive assessment and treatment concept for everyday life for children, and youths and adults with EB. The aim of a holistic concept is to provide a contribution to improving occupational performance and the quality of life for those affected.

In terms of content the following thematic priorities are covered:
- Therapeutic support of the early motor and perceptual development including the development of grasp and graphomotor skills
- Occupational therapy intervention focusing on independence in everyday life
- The functional treatment of the hands and feet of those with EB

The authors are aware that the combination of the paediatric and the functional areas of therapy is unusual. However, we believe that in view of the particular needs of people with EB, the functional approach used up till now in hand rehabilitation alone is not enough.

The variety of methods of intervention within occupational therapy offers many possibilities which can be goal-orientated for EB and so are brought together in this book.

It would not have been possible to produce this book without the support of our clients. With their experience they have contributed a great deal by giving us feedback on the different coping strategies in everyday situations. In this way it was possible for us to develop practical measures, which can be implemented easily. We would like to thank our clients for the numerous feedbacks out of their abundant treasure trove of experiences.

We are extremely grateful to *DEBRA Austria*, and in particular Dr. Rainer Riedl (Chairman, *DEBRA Austria*), for financing the project and thus making it possible. Most especially, our thanks go to Barbara Dissauer, research coordinator of *DEBRA Austria*. With her humorous, supportive and competent manner, she has led us through the ups and downs of the project.

Our gratitude goes also to the team of EB House Austria, above all Dr. Anja Diem who supported us wholeheartedly, and motivated us in times of need. We appreciate this extremely valuable teamwork very much. Dr. Rudolf Hametner and Walter Matschi contributed very significantly to the entire appearance of the book by providing pictures. Alexandra Waldhör contributed to the layout with her inventiveness and creative drawings.

We are indebted to assistant medical director Dr. Margret Burger-Rafael, Head of the EB Team of the University Clinic for Physical Medicine and Rehabilitation, for her support and technical advice and good cooperation. Astrid Fridrich, Dr. Andrea Wenger, Nicky Jessop and Ursula Costa, all experienced occupational therapists, gave us valuable recommendations and professional comments for the book. Marie Christin Pölzleitner provided excellent preparation in the form of her thesis 'Ergotherapie bei Epidermolysis bullosa in der Handrehabilitation' (Occupational Therapy for Clients with Epidermolysis Bullosa in Hand Rehabilitation) which we were able to build on.

We also thank Dr. Eva Maria Stöckler for her careful editing of the German manuscript and support in the formal realisation.

We extend a very big thank you to Prof. Patience Higman for the excellent translation of the book and the good cooperation during this intensive process.

Finally, I would like to thank my partner Christine and son Jakob, whose support and backing have always strengthen me and given me new vigour (Florian Prinz).

Contents

Contents

Contents

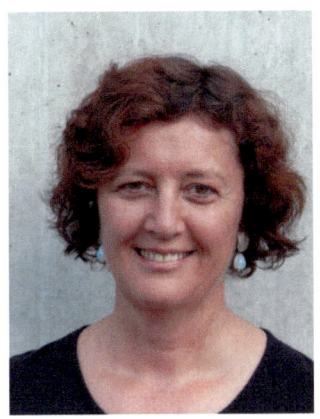

Hedwig Weiß MPhil.

Occupational therapist in the University Clinic for Physical Medicine and Rehabilitation at the State Hospital in Salzburg since 1994.

After training as an occupational therapist, Hedwig Weiß worked in geriatrics before studying the history of art at the University of Salzburg. Since then she has become an expert in hand therapy and has spent many years treating clients with epidermolysis bullosa, specialising in the provision of splints and functional treatment.

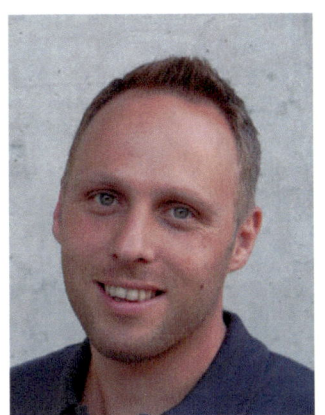

Florian Prinz

Occupational therapist in the University Clinic for Physical Medicine and Rehabilitation at the State Hospital in Salzburg and in his own paediatric occupational therapy practice.

He has run prevention projects to improve motor and perceptual functions in primary schools and has completed many continuing professional development courses in paediatric and hand therapy.

As a special needs educator he was the head of a kindergarten specialising in integration and Montessori pedagogics.

Florian Prinz has always been involved in early motor and perceptual development.

1 Epidermolysis Bullosa (EB) – the Condition

Hedwig Weiß and Florian Prinz

1.1   Definition

'**Bulla (lat.) f:** Blister; primary skin eruption; a cavity filled with liquid raised above the normal skin level; caused by a simple separation between the layers of the skin, usually only one chamber; at least 5 mm; differentiation is made between the localisation and the cause: subcorneal bulla (below the cornea), intra-epidermal bulla (in the epidermis), sub-epidermal bulla (between the epidermis and the corium) and acantholytic bulla (in the epidermis due to the breakup of the cell structures); bulla inflammatoris (inflammatory blister due to toxic noxa, inflammatory, allergic reactions, etc.), bulla mechanica (due to mechanical injury in epidermolysis), bulla actinica (due to exposure to the sun, e. g. hydroa vacciniforme), bulla spontanea (e. g. pemphigoid). Compare with efflorescence' (Pschyrembel 2012, p. 328).

'**Epidermolysis (; ; lys-*) f:** Separation and blister development in the dermoepidermal zones (e. g. e. bullosa acquisita, forms of e. bullosa hereditaria and bullous pemphigoid) or intra-epidermal (e. g. pemphigoid vulgaris)' (Pschyrembel 2012, p. 597).

Epidermolysis bullosa (EB): EB is a hereditary skin condition in which the skin of the affected person is liable to blistering. The skin can be as sensitive as the 'wing of a butterfly'.[1]

In this rare congenital condition there is a tendency for the skin to blister on account of minor injury. Sometimes, pressure or mild friction alone is sufficient to cause blistering. Depending on the form of the condition, this blistering can also affect the mucous membranes, especially in the mouth and the oesophagus.

The cause of this fragile skin and mucous membranes is a mutation in certain genes. The mutations are in the genes of the structural proteins of the dermoepidermal basement membrane zone (subepithelial). Normally, these structural proteins hold the layers of the skin together, but in this case they are deficient or defective in their function. Depending on the form, number and localisation, etc., there can be a very wide spectrum of possible clinical forms, which can vary from single blisters on the soles of the feet or palms of the hand to a generalisation over the whole body and the development of serious systemic complications. The clinical picture, progress, prognosis and course as well as the treatment can vary considerably. A causal treatment does not exist at present (cf. Laimer et al. 2008; Netzwerk EB 2009).

1.2   Pathology of EB

In principal, the classification of the three main forms of hereditary EB is done according to the level of blister formation in the skin.

---

1   Colloquially, children with EB are known as 'butterfly children'.

- **Epidermolysis bullosa simplex (EBS)** with fissure formation in the basal keratinocyte layer
- **Junctional EB (JEB)** with separation in the lamina lucida along the basement membrane
- **Dystrophic EB (DEB)** with dermolytic coherency dissociation below the lamina densa of the basement membrane (cf. Laimer et al. 2008; Netzwerk EB 2009)

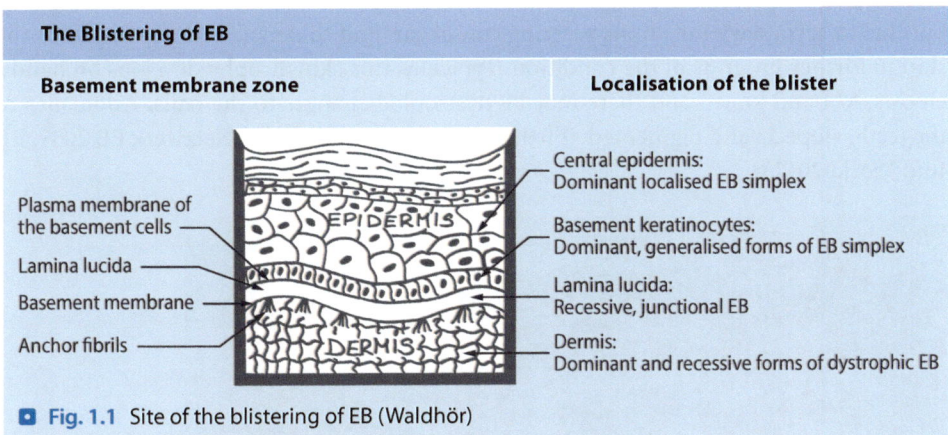

The Blistering of EB

Basement membrane zone	Localisation of the blister

Plasma membrane of the basement cells

Lamina lucida

Basement membrane

Anchor fibrils

Central epidermis: Dominant localised EB simplex

Basement keratinocytes: Dominant, generalised forms of EB simplex

Lamina lucida: Recessive, junctional EB

Dermis: Dominant and recessive forms of dystrophic EB

Fig. 1.1 Site of the blistering of EB (Waldhör)

In each of these main types there are many subdivisions (see p. 6–9).

Apart from the hereditary forms there is also an acquired form: EB acquisita. This is an autoimmune condition which is extremely rare (cf. Laimer et al. 2008).

1.2.1 EB Simplex (EBS)

EB simplex is the most common form of the condition. It is almost completely autosomal dominant inherited. The progressive form is usually mild; in childhood there is usually more blistering later, but the tendency remains lifelong. The healing of the blisters which develop intra-epidermally is normally without scarring or skin atrophy. Blistering happens mostly on the exposed areas, such as hands, feet, elbows, knees, etc., and is usually more during the summer months. Nails, mouth, mucous membrane and teeth are not affected, as can happen in other forms of EB (cf. Netzwerk EB 2009; EB Info World 2012).

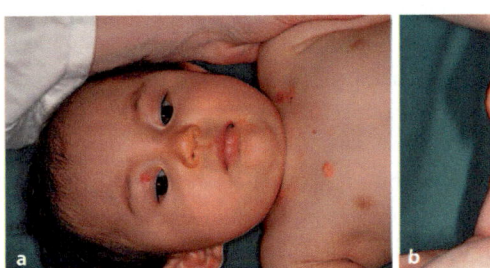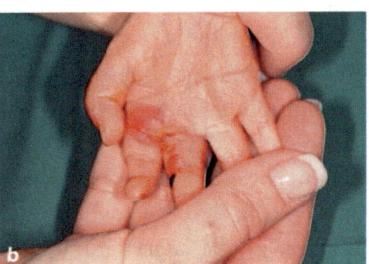

Fig. 1.2 **a** Infant with EBS (Hametner). **b** Hand of a child with EBS (Hametner)

1

1.2.2 Junctional EB (JEB)

This form of the condition is inherited autosomal recessively. Here there is a separation along the lamina lucida of the basement membrane, so that there is no cohesion between the epidermis and the dermis.

Depending on the severity of JEB, the progress can vary between minimal blistering and life-threatening limitations of skin function. Usually, the blisters heal without scarring, but due to secondary infections scarring can occur, and this may lead to atrophy of the skin in further progress of the condition. Typically, this skin atrophy develops on hands, elbows, feet and knees, and there may be dystrophic changes to the nails. Anomalies of the teeth, alopecia and pigmented (birthmark) may also occur (cf. Netzwerk EB 2009; EB Info World 2012).

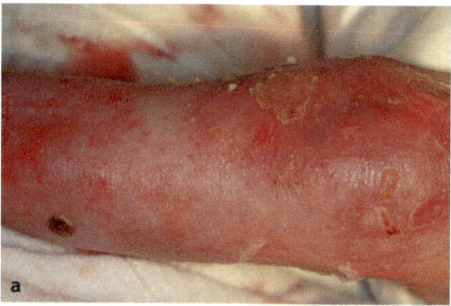
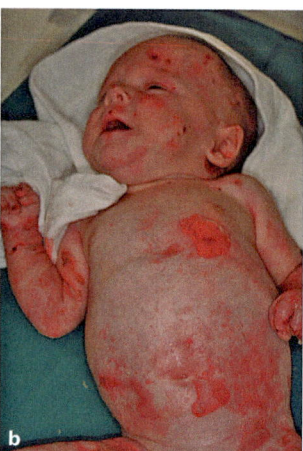

◘ Fig. 1.3 a Blisters on the leg of a child with JEB (Hametner) b Infant with JEB (Hametner)

1.2.3 Dystrophic EB (DEB)

This form of the condition is mostly inherited autosomal recessively. Usually there is scarring because the blistering is below the lamina densa, where the blood vessels and nerves are. Because of this the blisters can be very deep, contain blood and are painful. The blistering occurs as a result of injury, but it appears that sometimes it may be spontaneous. The clinical signs may vary considerably.

Scarring, milia (small white cysts) and nail dystrophy, and/or loss of nails are typical in this form of the condition. Usually, a flexor contracture of the fingers and a restriction of the abduction of the thumb develop.

Pseudosyndactyly may develop because the webbing grows between the fingers and toes; these may even go so far that the fingers and toes become mitten-like. Furthermore, there are often mutilations of the fingers and toes. The real cause of the pseudosyndactyly and mutilations are yet unknown.

The mucous membranes (especially in the mouth, the gastrointestinal and the urogenital tracts) are also affected in DEB.

The severity of the progress varies according to the subgroup from mild (usually in the dominantly inherited form) to a completely dependent state with a reduced life expectancy (RDEB severe generalised; Hallopeau-Siemens).

Further complications can be deformity of the teeth, defective hair growth on the head, anaemia, a tendency to squamous cell carcinoma (after early adolescence) and delayed growth (cf. Netzwerk EB 2009; EB Info World 2012; Pschyrembel 2012).

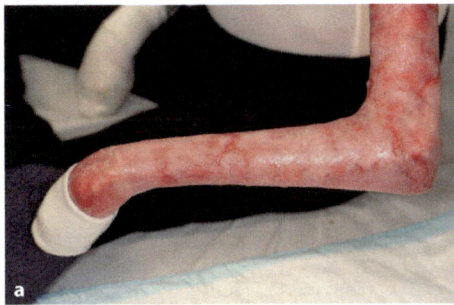 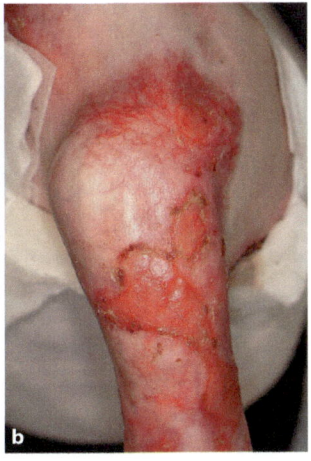

◘ Fig. 1.4 **a** Arm of a child with DEB (Hametner). **b** Child with DEB (Hametner)

1.3 The Most Common Sub-Types and Their Signs and Symptoms

Main form	Most common sub-types	Inheritance	Mutation shown in gene for	Signs and symptoms
EB simplex (EBS) Blistering due to cytolysis of basal keratin cells	EBS-localised (Weber-Cockayne) (EBS-loc)	AD	Keratin 5,14	Blisters, erosions, mainly palmar and plantar; mostly in the summer
	EBS-generalised, other (Koebner) (EBS-gen other)	AD	Keratin 5,14	Blisters, erosions, generalised on all extremities
	EBS-Dowling-Meara (EBS-DM)	AD	Keratin 5,14	Blisters, erosions, granulation tissue generalised; palmoplantar hyperkeratosis, nail dystrophy, atrophic scarring; includes the oral mucosa
	Recessive EBS (very rare)	AR	Keratin 14	Blisters and erosions generalised; palmoplantar hyperkeratosis, nail dystrophy, atrophic scarring
	EBS-Ogna (very rare)	AD	Plectin	Blisters, erosions, nail dystrophy
	EBS-muscular dystrophy (EBS-MD) (very rare)	AR	Plectin	Blisters, erosions, nail dystrophy; progressive muscular dystrophy with onset between birth and 4th decade
Junctional EB (JEB) Junctional splitting of the lamina lucida	JEB-Herlitz (JEB-H)[2]	AR	Laminin-332	Blistering with atrophic scarring, chronic granulating erosions, dystrophy of the nail bed, loss of nails, oral mucosal fragility, enamel hypoplasia of the teeth; airway granulation tissue and scarring; failure to thrive; death usual in first year of life
	JEB-non-Herlitz (JEB-nH)	AR	Laminin-332, Type XVII collagen	Blisters, erosions, granulation tissue, atrophic scars, scarring alopecia, loss of nails
	JEB with pyloric atresia (JEB-PA)	AR	Integrin α6β4	Usually severe blistering, erosions, granulation tissue; congenital pyloric atresia (obstruction of the lower part of the stomach, the pylorus)

2 Approximately 90% of the affected children die in the first year of life (cf. Yan et al. 2007).

Dystrophic EB (DEB) Dermolytic splitting below the lamina densa			
Dominant DEB (DDEB)	AD	Type VII collagen	Blistering, erosions, milia; atrophic scars (especially on the extremities), nail dystrophy and loss of nails
Recessive DEB severe generalised (Hallopeau-Siemens) (RDEB-sev gen)	AR	Type VII collagen	Blistering, erosions, granulation tissue; atrophic scars, scarring alopecia, loss of nails, scarring deformities of hands and feet (pseudosyndactyly, contractures); oral mucosal fragility and scarring and microstomia
RDEB generalised other (non-Hallopeau-Siemens) (RDEB-gen other)	AR	Type VII collagen	Blisters, erosions, granulation tissue, atrophic scars, nail loss and dystrophy; oral mucosa fragility and scarring

(cf. Fine et al. 2008; Laimer et al. 2003)

1.4 The Most Common Cutaneous and Extracutaneous Complications

Usually in the case of:	Cutaneous complications		Treatment strategies (abbreviated)
RDEB-sev gen, RDEB-gen other, sometimes JEB-nH and DDEB	Squamous cell carcinoma	Often multiple, aggressive behaviour, often poor response to chemo- and radiotherapy	Careful and constant inspection of clinically suspicious and non-healing wounds; early excision and operative intervention
All sub-types, especially JEB-nH	Pigmented lesions	Very large light to dark brown or black moles or naevi; often joining with a blister; become lighter with age; clinical and histopathological parallels with characteristics of melanomas, however no known malignant development	Regular inspection; if necessary histological examination of suspicious lesions (even multiple)
RDEB	Melanoma	Increased risk in childhood even without previous lesions	Regular inspection; if necessary histological examination of suspicious lesions (even multiple)
RDEB-sev gen; seldom JEB, DDEB and EBS	Pseudosyndactyly	Mitten deformity of fingers and toes; atrophy of the digits, contractures of the thumb, interphalangeal and metacarpophalangeal joints; deformities and limited or complete loss of function of the hands and feet; high tendency to postoperative relapse (repeat operations required on average every 5 years)	Surgical intervention, physical therapy (including night splinting)
Usually in the case of:	Extracutaneous manifestations		
JEB, DEB	Teeth and gastrointestinal tract	Enamel hypoplasia (JEB), tooth dysplasia, excessive caries, microstomia (small mouth) (DEB), early loss of teeth; oesophageal and anal strictures (DEB), dysphagia (DEB), chronic constipation, painful defecation; failure to thrive	Careful dental hygiene, orthodentistry, repeated dilatation of the oesophagus (DEB), diet advice, regulation of bowel movement; gastrostomy

JEB, RDEB (rarely)	Respiratory tract	Oedema of the mucous membranes, blisters, erosions, scarring; hoarseness, laryngeal stenosis, acute respiratory obstruction	Tracheostomy, corticosteroids, antibiotics
JEB, RDEB	Eyes	Corneal erosion, scarring of the cornea, symblepharon (adhesion of one or both eyelids to the eyeball), electropium (lack of tear fluid as a result of adhesions), blepharitis (inflammation of the eyelids), lacrimal duct stenosis, impaired vision	Moistening eye drops, analgesia, surgery
JEB, DEB	Urogenital tract	Dysuria, haematuria, stenosis, obstruction; vesicoureteral reflux, hydronephrosis, renal hypertension, urosepsis, glomerulonephritis, amyloidosis, renal failure	Regular blood pressure and urinalysis, avoid instrumentation unless strictly necessary; catheterisation, cystoscopy, urethral dilatation, meatotomy, haemodialysis, peritoneal dialysis
All serious forms	Metabolism and general symptoms	Loss of nutrients and proteins due to the denuded areas of skin, catabolic metabolism with increased need for calories; nutritional deficiencies; growth retardation, impaired wound healing and general health, repeated infections, chronic anaemia	Optimisation of oral nutrition; supportive replacement therapy; gastrostomy feeding

(cf. Fine, Mellerio 2009; Laimer et al. 2008)

1.5   Diagnosis

The importance of the diagnosis of this condition is because the changes at a molecular level correlate with the symptoms, progress and prognosis. The exact diagnosis enables a prediction as to the fate of the affected person and makes it possible to plan an adaptive treatment strategy to give the best possible quality of life.

The diagnostic procedure begins with an exact case history and clinical examination. The family history is especially important to determine whether such a blister forming skin condition is known in the family and whether consanguinity exists (cf. Netzwerk EB 2009).

Apart from taking the case history and clinical examination, two special diagnostic procedures are used:
- Antigen mapping
- Mutation analysis

1.6   Therapy

In recent years, there has been intensive research into gene therapy with the aim of finding a causative cure. Although substantial progress has been made, only a purely symptomatic treatment is possible at present.

Such treatment includes the prevention or reduction of blistering by using protective measures in daily life. Further afflictions may be reduced by using an adequately adapted nutrition; sometimes a percutaneous endoscopic gastrostomy (PEG) tube is necessary. Professional wound management can also be alleviating (cf. Laimer et al. 2008).

Surgical intervention may sometimes be necessary to release webbing of the fingers and toes (pseudosyndactyly). Following this operation, occupational therapy (OT) enables the highest possible mobility and independence. The complexity of the condition requires an interdisciplinary team.

2 Motor Development in Early Childhood

Florian Prinz

EB is a serious condition, which depending on its form, influences many parts of the body. Until now, occupational therapy (OT) intervention has usually concentrated on hand function, which may be extremely limited, especially in JEB and DEB. The overall motor development has probably been largely neglected because of all the other problems.

It is easy to understand that blisters and wounds covering the body have a significant influence on early physical movement and can limit a child's exploration of its environment. Considering the value of this early basic experience and the influence on further development, it deserves greater therapeutic attention.

Thinking along these lines, intervention for children with EB has been extended beyond hand and grip function to include the complete motor and perceptual development.

2.1   Motor Development Screening

It has proved expedient to carry out gross motor development screening in children with EB aged between 18 months and 4 years. Only with increasing age of the children is the emphasis gradually shifted to the assessment of the tactile, vestibular and proprioceptive senses (see p. 29).

The milestones of motor development in early childhood as described, for example, by Largo (2007) can be used for orientation. The very wide range of ages at which early motor development manifests itself must, however, always be taken into consideration.

As a further support tool, a parental questionnaire on early motor development (see p. 18) can be used and the basic motor development steps and environmental exploration behaviour of the child recorded. The questionnaire has been especially adjusted for children with EB and enables therapists to gain an overall picture of possible developmental delays or deficits. This knowledge can then be used in planning the intervention.

2.1.1   Typical Development of Motor Ability

3–6 Months

Head control: At the age of 3 months an infant can raise his/her head to look ahead while lying face down. The child supports him-/herself on the elbows/forearms and begins to look at and follow objects. At 6 months the baby can turn his/her head to either side and look up and down while in this position.

A bimanual grip is first possible at approximately 3 to 5 months.

Active rolling over/support on hands when lying face down: Between 3 and 7 months infants roll over, first from their backs or fronts onto their sides. Then they roll from their fronts onto their backs, and finally from their backs onto their fronts (cf. Largo 2007).

An important milestone in the development is firstly the support on the forearms at approximately 6 months, then support on the hands while lying face down (like a 'press-up'). In this position the infant can raise most of the thorax away from the surface he/she is lying on and so is able to see a full 360°. This is important for the development of the visual–spatial perception as well as the later positioning of the head, shoulders and trunk when sitting at a table to play (Nacke 2005).

6–10 Months

Creeping: Initially, only the arms are used; the infant supports him-/herself on his/her elbows or hands and pulls the body forwards. Later the legs are used as well, and soon after that it becomes alternating – this is known as 'creeping'.

Crawling: Infants mostly begin to rock in a quadruped position; this trains the muscles and the stability in preparation for holding an upright position. This is followed by crawling.

Sitting: Once an infant can roll over 360° and get onto his/her hands and knees from a prone position, he/she soon learns to sit up and lie down again. While sitting, the hands are free to play. The infant can participate more actively in his/her environment.

10–24 Months (Second Year)

Pulling up with the help of furniture/standing: From about 9–15 months the infant uses furniture to pull him-/herself up into a standing position – then he/she begins to take his/her first steps sideways along the furniture using it for support.

Walking: This stage of development spans a very wide age range. While some toddlers can walk freely at 9 months, others can only do this at about 18 or 20 months although their development is perfectly normal. This depends largely on how fast this skill develops and it cannot really be influenced by practice. Most children take their first steps at about 13 to 14 months.

Walking, however, does not complete the motor development. In the beginning the toddler walks with his/her feet wide apart to compensate for the lack of stability. At this point the pelvic girdle is not yet fully upright in relation to gravity. The arms are often held bent at the elbows and are used for support and to hold on to supports; only later do they swing at the sides in rhythm with the gait and can be used more freely. In the next step, the child begins to walk by rolling the foot from heel to toe. Change of direction is achieved more easily and the speed can be varied to suit different conditions. Now the toddler can push or pull a wheeled toy. He/she learns to squat down from standing and pick things up from the floor. At the age of 2 years the toddler can stop at will and stand still. Running so that both feet are momentarily off the ground is not yet rhythmical (Nacke 2005; Becker, Steding-Albrecht 2006; Largo 2007).

Throwing a ball: From about 13 to 18 months a toddler can throw but does so aimlessly. The fun of running after the ball is more important to him/her. At 24 months the toddler is not yet able to kick a ball in a specific direction; he/she runs into the rolling ball without being able to take any conscious action (Becker, Steding-Albrecht 2006).

2

In general: Recent studies (Largo 2007; Pikler, Tardos 2001) of the locomotion development of healthy children show that the development of the early movement is a much more wide-ranging process than was previously realised. The majority of children develop as described above. Some children miss out specific phases or, for example move forward on their bottom instead of crawling (see Fig. 2.1).

The age range of development is also much larger than had previously been described. Practice cannot influence the start of the early child motor function, but the finer development of an existing function is dependent on how much it is put to use (Largo 2007).

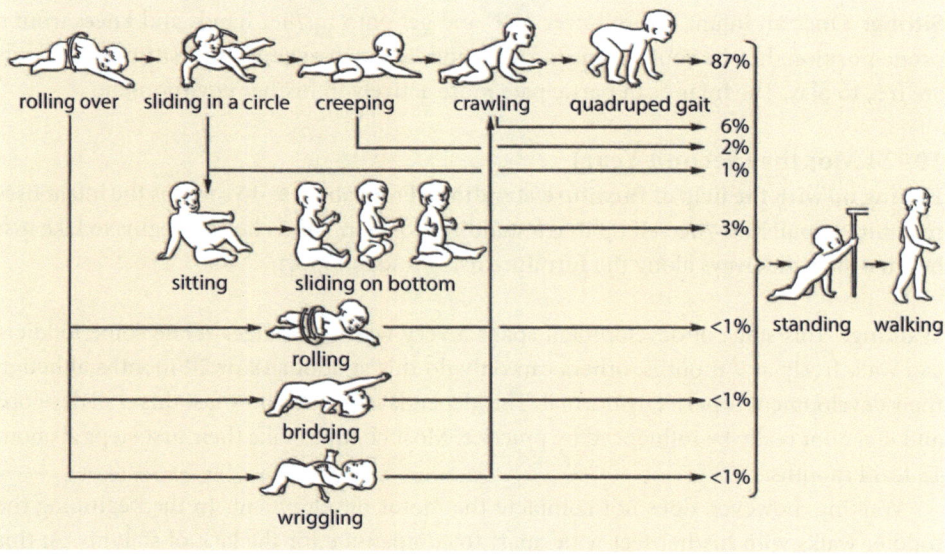

◘ **Fig. 2.1** New presentation of locomotion (© Largo 2007, p. 130)

24–36 Months (Third Year)

At the start of the third year the motor skills are being tried out and improved or refined; this may result in many falls at the beginning. By the end of the third year the movements are more fluid and controlled. The toddler walks safely and independently, carries things around and climbs on chairs and other objects, seeking a challenge. Going down stairs is achieved step by step initially but, by the end of the third year, can be done by alternating the feet. The child enjoys balancing on things; doing so on a beam as narrow as 20 cm is possible. He/she enjoys swinging and throws large balls with both hands. Catching is usually more coincidental. By the end of the third year a child learns to ride a tricycle (Becker, Steding-Albrecht 2006).

36–48 Months (Fourth Year)

The child plays on simple apparatus in the playground without help. He/she can aim a distance of 1–2 m successfully when throwing and a ball can be caught at chest height with the arms. The child can stand on one leg for about 2 s and can crawl under a gymnastic bench and do a summersault. Jumping over a rope is only possible with both legs together at first. Overall, the quality of movement improves and the muscle tone matches the task better.

48–60 Months (Fifth Year)

A scooter, tricycle or other pedal toy can be steered safely; the child is able to pedal and steer at the same time. A hindrance can be avoided. The child can jump 30–50 cm forwards from standing and can jump over a rope with the feet singly. In the playground he/she climbs and plays on a gym apparatus a great deal. He/she can stand on one leg for 3–4 s (Becker, Steding-Albrecht 2006).

2.1.2 Assessment of Children with EB

It is best to provide an opportunity with suitable play equipment where the child can play and exercise according to his/her age, in as normal a manner as possible so that he/she can be observed and analysed. A room with space for freedom of movement is best. To minimise the risk of falling or bumping there should be little furniture, and what there is should not have sharp corners. Gymnastic mats, for example from Airex®, provide a good surface for simple balancing or ball games, etc. because they reduce pressure on painful blisters. For crawling or other movements on the floor, such mats are unsuitable because there is too much friction, which causes the development of blisters. Smooth parquet flooring or firm mats with a smooth covering are more suitable.

Before starting the child should be inspected for blisters and open wounds. If removal of bandaging is painful and complicated, then the parents should be consulted. It must be taken into consideration that pain on particularly prominent places such as knees, elbows, abdomen, instep and soles of the feet can lead to avoidance tactics in certain movements or tasks.

What to Observe

Sitting

- How does the child get into the sitting position?
  How does the child sit (straighten up from the hips, trunk, head) | stability in sitting | can the child vary the sitting positions | use of arms while sitting | hand–hand coordination | eye–hand coordination?

Locomotion on the floor (e. g. crawling after a ball)

- How does the child move (creep, slide on the bottom, crawl | alternating | does the child show signs of relieving postures or one-sided weight bearing)?
- How does he/she change position? (transfer from sitting to locomotion)

- How does he/she cope with obstacles? (motor planning | position of the head and extremities while crawling under obstacles – proprioception)

Transfer from floor to upright
- Does the child change to kneeling to pull him-/herself up on furniture?
- Or, has the child developed an alternative method to get into an upright position (e. g.: from quadruped position | pushing up with his/her bottom against a wall)?

Walking
- Gait (weight bearing on the feet | relieving postures | positioning of the feet, the hips, the head | width of gait | stability | postural security | arm swinging | transfer of weight from heel to forefoot | overcoming obstacles | stopping intentionally | change of direction | picking up objects from the floor)

Going up and down stairs
- Step by step or alternating?
- Holding on or not?

Jump off the ground with both feet
- Is jumping off with both feet possible (from the floor | from a mat or trampoline)?
- Timing, coordination of the legs and arms when jumping
- Stability on landing

Balancing course
Walking on a soft mat, on a balance board or on soft cushions or sandbags
- Balance, stability, compensatory movement
- Standing upright against the pull of gravity with increasing need to keep balance when, for example, on an unstable surface such as a foam mat. Does the child show excessive compensatory movement?
- Speed of locomotion
- Quality of locomotion

Climbing on wallbars or a ladder
- Position of hips, trunk and head while climbing
- Climbing step by step or alternating
- Proprioception (conscious positioning of extremities without visual control)
- Coordination of the upper and lower extremities
- Opposition of the thumb (so long as there is no hand deformity) when holding the bars
- Achieving height (careful | frightened | confident)
- Judging own abilities
- Judging danger

Throwing and catching a ball
- Stability when catching and throwing
- Timing and hand–hand coordination when catching
- Ability to aim and adjust force when throwing

Riding a Bobbycar (car to sit on and propel with feet on the ground)/tricycle
- Can the child hold and use the steering wheel or steering stick in spite of possible limitations of the hands (mutilations and pseudosyndactyly caused by DEB may make it difficult or impossible)?
- Is steering done by lifting and turning the vehicle or by conscious use of the steering mechanism?
- How does the child cope with obstacles?
- Can the child pedal and steer a tricycle simultaneously (from the age of 5 years)?

2.1.3   Parental Questionnaire Focusing on the Early Motor Development

2

Parental questionnaire focusing on the early motor development
For children with epidermolysis bullosa (EB)

Motor development

Motor ability	Age in months	Were (are) there any EB-specific problems or difficulties?
Raise head and upper trunk while prone		
Roll from tummy to back		
Roll from back to tummy		
Creep		
Crawl		
Sit		
Pull up to standing on furniture		
Stand without support		
Walk without support		
Walk downstairs		
Walk upstairs		

Early child exploration

The child explored/s his/her environment using:				
	Age in months	yes	no	If no, is there a reason due to EB?
Mouth		O	O	
Hands		O	O	
Eyes		O	O	
Feet		O	O	

2.2 Results from Motor Development Screening

The authors describe what is known to date from clinical experience concerning the motor and perceptual development (see p. 33). Summing it up, there were delays of varying degrees in the early motor development in nearly all the assessed children. Children with EBS, JEB and DEB were screened.

Locomotion on the Floor

The reports from the parents show that the majority of children with EB avoid the prone position as infants and later also avoid creeping and crawling. It can be interpreted that this avoidance is due to the painful blistering and injury on the abdomen, elbows, knees, thighs, insteps or hands (see Fig. 2.2a,b and Fig. 2.3a,b). These areas experience particular strain in the prone position and when creeping and crawling. The friction causes increased blistering, whereas pressure has a smaller negative effect and, as a rule, can be tolerated more easily.

Many children with EB slide around on their bottoms as an alternative to crawling (3 % of all typically developing children do this), as this causes the least blistering and pain. From this position locomotion is possible (children explore their environment by sliding), also the arms are free to explore, but later the transfer to an upright position is physiologically more difficult.

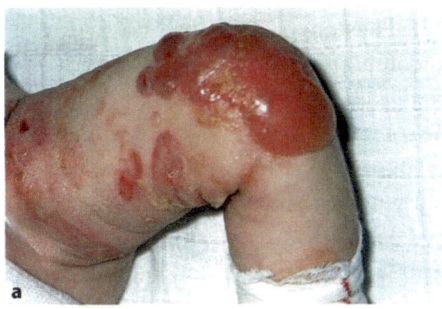
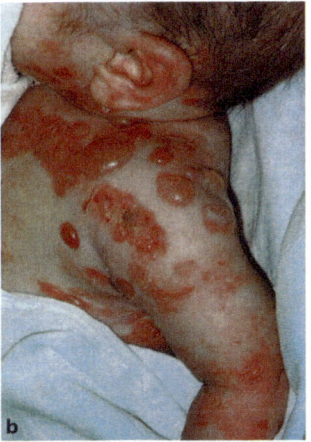

◘ Fig. 2.2a,b Blisters on the extremities and trunk (DEBRA Austria)

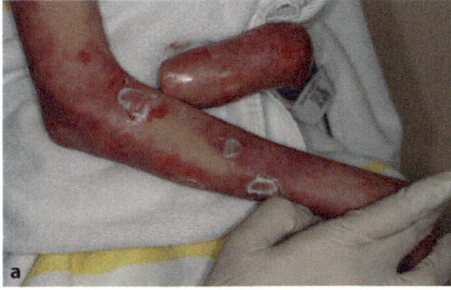
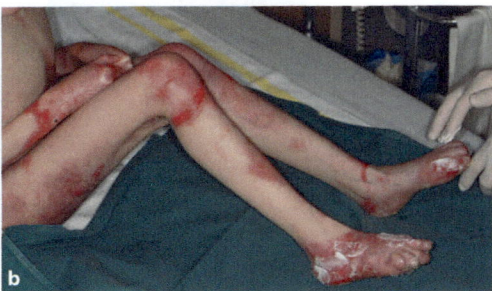

◘ Fig. 2.3a,b Blisters on the extremities (Hametner)

2

Sitting

Observations to date show that children with EB sit unsupported later than typically developing children (between 7 and 10 months). The delayed development of active sitting can be understood when realising that this position is usually achieved from the all fours, which is often avoided by the children because of the painful load on the knees.

Once active sitting is achieved, many children with EB remain passively in this position for a long time because a transfer again causes pain.

Transfer from Floor to an Upright Position

It is necessary to transfer to the knees when pulling up on furniture from sitting; this causes pain, in particular for children with JEB and DEB, and so it is avoided. This partly explains the generally late start of standing and walking.

Some children develop compensatory strategies to be able to change position. For example, the transfer from the prone position to sitting without bending the knees but by straddling the legs, as in doing the splits, has been observed. Some children manage to stand by sliding up against walls with their bottoms and backs.

Pushing up against Gravity/Walking

There is a delay in comparison with their peers in unsupported standing and walking, shown by children with JEB and DEB (based on the knowledge that unsupported walking in typically developing children is achieved, at the latest, by 20 months). Further many children stand out due to poor quality of movement, poor postural control and a lack of variation of locomotion. In rare cases unsupported walking is not achieved.

When standing and walking, blistering on the soles of the feet cause pain, which children try to avoid either by only using part of the foot or by spreading the load to the complete sole and so avoiding the heel-to-toe motion. Pseudosyndactyly, especially in the area of the big toe, can also influence stability (see Fig. 2.4a,b). The parents of affected children have reported that the children avoided moving about independently and attempting an upright position, and wanted to be carried for a long time.

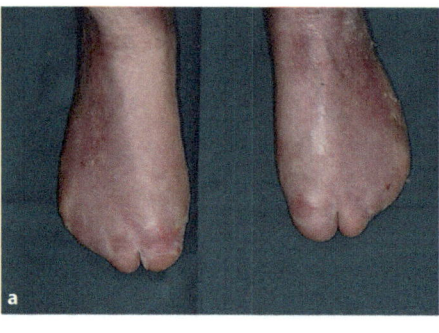
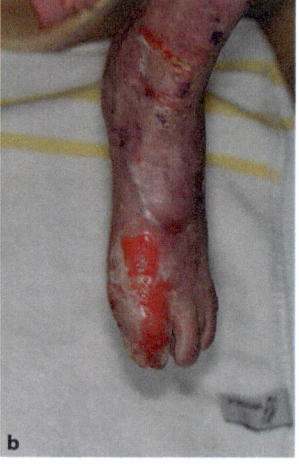

◘ Fig. 2.4 a Pseudosyndactyly of the toes (Hametner). **b** Blistering on the big toe (Hametner)

The gait of many children with EB often reveals poor position of the lower extremity (arches of the feet, ankles, knees), insufficient righting of the pelvis and a wide instable pace. Further a poor righting of the head can be observed; this is explained by the poor position of the feet linking to the pelvis and trunk (from caudal to cranial). Apart from that there is a noticeable asymmetrical pattern because of relieving postures and slow pace.

The cause of this posture pattern, which has often been observed, is partly due to the relieving postures and partly a sign of the late and immature motor development. Many children have a gait similar to those learning to walk, even when they are much older (lack of tipping of the pelvis, arms in readiness for a fall, wide gait) (see Fig. 2.5a,b).

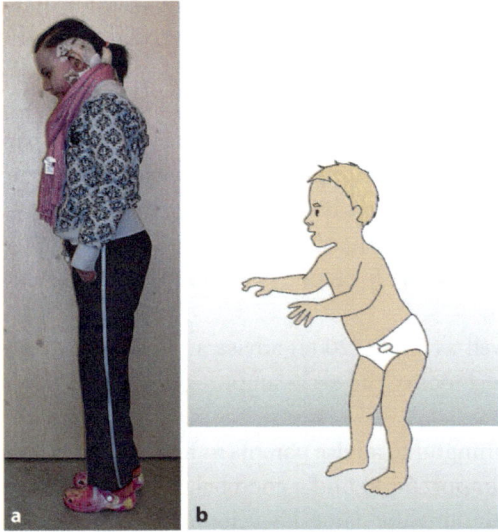

☐ **Fig. 2.5** Comparison of uprighting and posture in standing. **a** Child with DEB in the described posture (Hametner). **b** Still incomplete standing posture at 1 year (eXakt PR)

Putz (1999) writes that scarring in the neck and shoulder areas can be the cause of limitations to movement in those affected by EB (see Fig. 2.6). There can also be an imbalance of muscles because of scarring around the ankles, knees, shoulders and elbows.

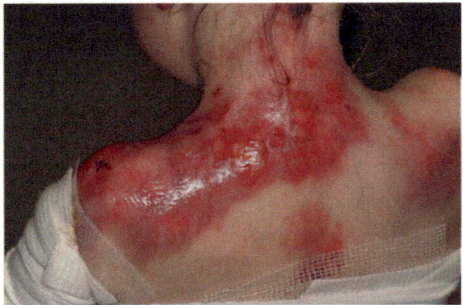

☐ **Fig. 2.6** Scarring in the neck region (Hametner)

2

Considering the frequently observed posture and locomotion patterns described above, it can be concluded that they are the cause of the development of the limitations of movement and muscle imbalance. The flexion pattern of the hips, knees and neck resulting from a poor posture is increased by the pull of the scarring. The child is thus 'fixed' in this pattern.

2.3   Occupational Therapy

2.3.1   Advising Parents

Parents have an understandable tendency to overprotect their children with EB due to the worry of injury and blistering. There is often little confidence placed in the children with regard to mobility, and they are not always encouraged to try things. Many (but not all) children with EB anyway show a rather cautious retiring behaviour, and this tendency is often reinforced by parents. It leads to passiveness and a lack of movement. To date parents have been advised by doctors to be protective so as to prevent too much scarring and the resulting contractures early on. Many children are carried for a long time, and even when they can sit freely, the parents hand them toys. The children are thus not prompted to change position actively and so learn the transfers from one position to another and to become mobile.

Today Burger-Rafael (2005, 2009) as well as Diem (2009) advise a rethinking of this protective attitude and emphasise the importance of the early support of motor development for children with EB.

From the OT aspect, it is therefore meaningful to advise parents to help their children from the start of motor development. It is important to find a good balance here between preventing injury and blistering, and encouraging the natural development of movement of the child. The following section describes methods to assist motor development, which parents can carry out at home.

2.3.2   OT Intervention Focusing on the Early Motor Development

According to current knowledge, early OT intervention is meaningful in the area of motor development, particularly for infants with DEB and, depending on the severity, JEB and EBS.

The question of relevance to daily life, which is always in the forefront of OT intervention, is answered by the fact that the specific limitations of EB on the motor development have a significant influence on competence of the children in their everyday routines. A passive attitude to movement prevents the children from exploring their environment and surroundings. It restricts learning about three-dimensional space through overcoming obstacles as well as experiencing the vertical position in sitting and standing. Reduced motor abilities hinder the children in mobility and independence, and make the participation in games with others of the same age, or the integration in a playgroup or gymnastics in preschool nursery difficult.

OT Intervention

The interventions described here should be seen as examples and need to be adjusted from child to child to ensure the meaningfulness and usefulness:

- To encourage the often-avoided prone position and exploration while the body is supported on the forearms, a soft insulating material (e. g. viscoelastic foam, often known as 'memory foam') can be added to the outer layers of bandaging on the front, the elbows and the knees. To minimise friction while creeping and crawling, the wrists may also be bandaged.
- It is advisable to use mats which are not too soft and have a smooth surface, to minimise the friction when creeping and crawling.
- If the mat is too soft, it gives the child an unstable base, which increases the demands of balancing and the child may be unable to cope. Using the usual gymnastic mats has shown that they provide a good insulation for specific balancing exercises, but for learning to creep and crawl they provide too much resistance and friction because of the 'soft-grip' surface.
- Such play apparatus as coloured balls, balloons, glowing balls and rattling eggs are especially good to encourage creeping and crawling because of their high-challenging character and because their mobility encourages chasing them. In addition, it has been shown that there is a much higher willingness to move when the internal motivation is encouraged and the play is fun. The subjective pain appears to be lower when the situation is fun orientated.
- The use of therapy balls (see Fig. 2.7) and padded therapy rolls offer protection of the trunk and minimises the pressure on hands and knees; being on hands and knees is a prerequisite for crawling.

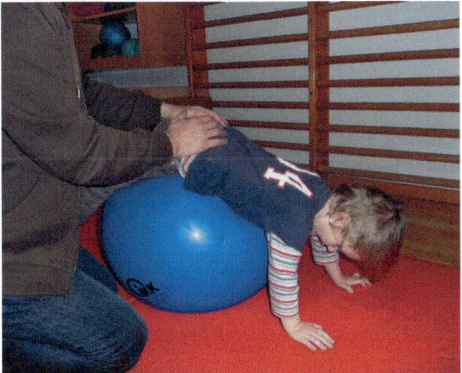

☐ Fig. 2.7 Child supporting itself on its hands while using a therapy ball

2

- Elbow and knee protectors made of neoprene (see Fig. 2.8) can be an added help in minimising pressure and friction.

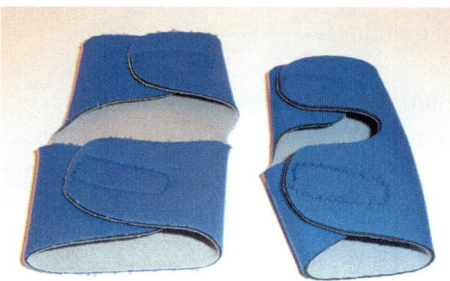

■ **Fig. 2.8** Elbow and knee protectors made of neoprene

- When the sitting position cannot be achieved actively from all fours because of blisters on the knees, it may be possible to learn to get there via a side-sitting method (see Fig. 2.9). That way the knees are protected, but the child must use elbows (elbow protectors should be used).

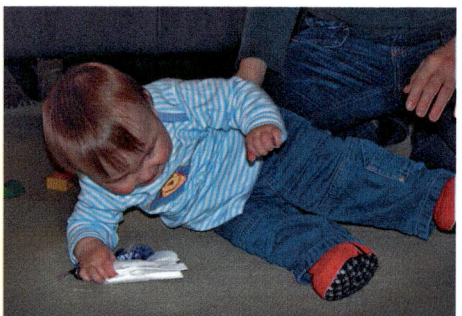

■ **Fig. 2.9** Sitting up via the side-sitting method

- In both therapy and at home it is best to have a room that provides space to move freely with little furniture, no sharp corners (they can be suitably covered) and no carpets to trip over, thus lowering the danger of injury. Wall-to-wall carpeting is soft, but it causes serious friction for creeping and crawling.
- As therapy progresses small obstacles to overcome can be incorporated. Soft play areas (see Fig. 2.10) made of covered foam offer a variety of movement and perceptual possibilities. At home such play areas can be created quite easily by using cushions, sandbags and pieces of foam or mattresses.
  In this way balance and locomotion planning are trained. Crawling through an obstacle (e. g. foam elements like a tunnel) requires an exact positioning of the extremities and makes it possible to experience three-dimensional space.

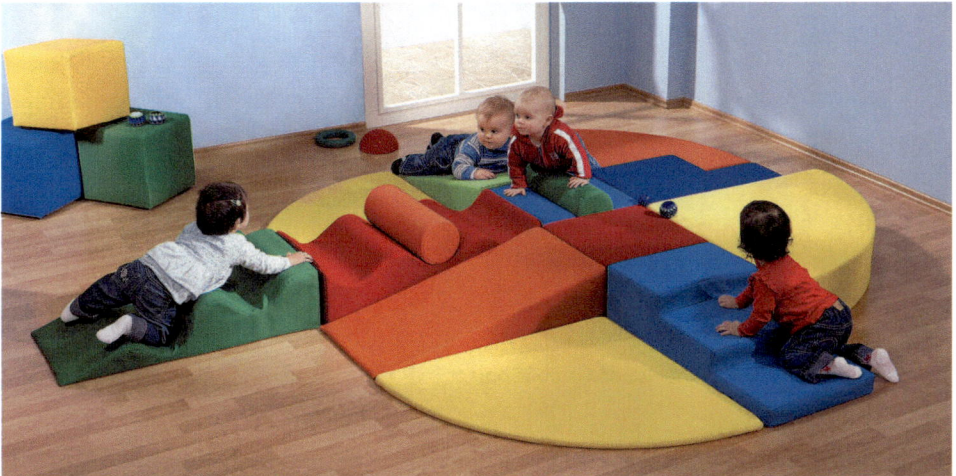

◘ **Fig. 2.10** Soft play area made of covered foam (Wehrfritz)

- As described, many children have difficulties transferring independently from the knees to standing. As compensation, getting up from side sitting via a quadruped position may help (see Fig. 2.11 a,b). In that way there is no pressure on the knees.

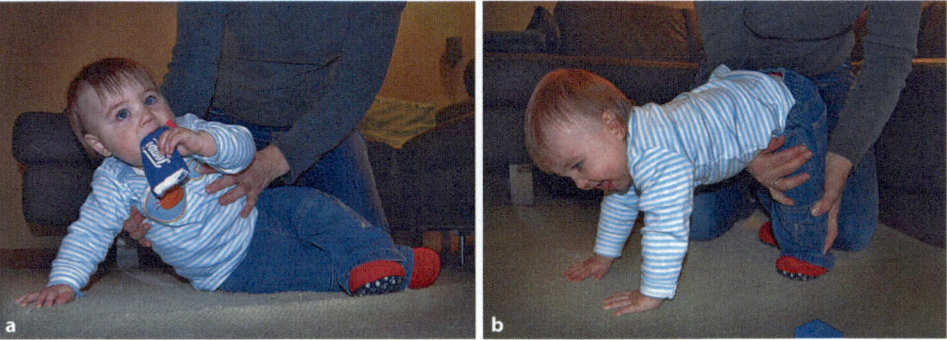

◘ **Fig. 2.11a,b** Transfer from side sitting via quadruped position to standing

- To support standing and walking, slippers with sheepskin linings, padded with gel or inlays of viscoelastic foam may be used.
- When walking unsupported is still unsafe, mobile objects such as a stool or doll pram (weighted) can help. The child can hold on and push the object forwards (see Fig. 2.12).

2

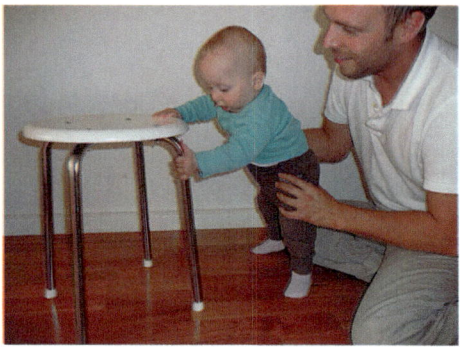

◘ **Fig. 2.12** Walking with the use of a mobile object

- Inflatable softballs, soft foam balls or balloons may be used for ball games.
- Climbing on wall bars can be painful because of the pressure on only part of the soles of the feet; wearing padded shoes spreads the pressure over a wider space and so reduces pain.
  Also padding the bars where the feet are placed can provide relief. The complete bar should not be padded as that increases the diameter of the individual bar and that may make it even harder to grip.
- Sheepskin on the saddle or sitting area of riding cars and tricycles can reduce pressure there. Rocking horses and similar toys may be so adapted (see Fig. 2.13a). If gripping the steering wheel is limited or not possible because of hand deformity, it makes sense to make appropriate grip adaptations (see Fig. 2.13b).
- Other ideas for locomotion for toddlers can be found in Chap. 6.2.2 from p. 80.

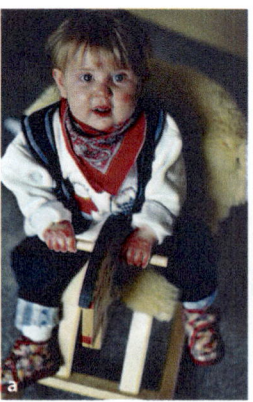
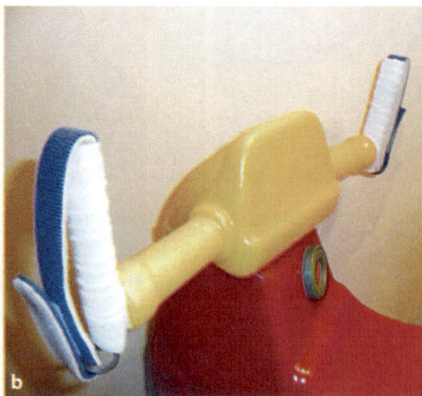

◘ **Fig. 2.13 a,b** Adaptations for rocking horse and tricycle. **a** Sheepskin for a soft seat (Hametner). **b** Grip adaptation

3 Treatment of the Tactile, Vestibular and Proprioceptive Perception

Florian Prinz

At the beginning of the therapeutic work with EB affected children, the question arises whether, and if so when, the condition influences the tactile, vestibular and proprioceptive perception.

3.1 Hypotheses Concerning Perception

Hypothesis 1

Hypothesis 1 assumes that the specific restrictions of the condition affect perception and motor functions, for example due to damage to the receptors in the skin and due to the lack of experience because of the limited possibilities for exploration.

This subject has been largely ignored in the small amount of literature available. Putz (1999) surmises that there is a loss of the tactile sense because of the large areas of skin damage on the soles of the feet and attributes the loss of equilibrium in walking to the same cause.

Hypothesis 2

Hypothesis 2 assumes that the sensory processing at a central level in children with EB is also affected, thus causing difficulties in amplifying, inhibiting, filtering, comparison and association of sensory information.

There is no mention of this subject in the usual textbooks on EB.

To clarify the meaning of tactile, vestibular and proprioceptive perception, they are defined here, and an explanation of the sensory processing disorders from the standpoint of sensory integration therapy is given.

3.1.1 The Relevance of Tactile, Vestibular and Proprioceptive Perception to Child Development

Ayres, the founder of sensory integration therapy, considered tactile, vestibular and proprioceptive perception essential to child development and to fundamental neural organisation (cf. Becker, Steding-Albrecht 2006). These areas of perception form the basis for the development of more advanced abilities. The tactile, proprioceptive and vestibular systems are especially important in newborns because of the role they have in taking in information from the environment. Contact with the mother is through the skin. When being carried, held and moved the infant experiences proprioceptive and vestibular input. Adequate processing of the tactile, proprioceptive and vestibular stimuli is one of the basics for the development of body scheme, posture and vestibular abilities, muscle tone, coordination, motor planning, attention span, eye movements etc.

The senses of taste, smell, vision and hearing together with the information from the tactile, proprioceptive and vestibular systems enable the development of higher abilities, such as dexterity for writing or handicrafts, understanding language, ability to speak, concentration, learning to read and write as well as self-confidence etc. (cf. Ayres 2002).

The tactile, vestibular and proprioceptive perception is understood to have a basic and an integrating effect. Problems with learning and adaptive behaviour are therefore attributed to inadequate processing of the tactile, vestibular and proprioceptive information (cf. Becker, Steding-Albrecht 2006).

Definition and Development of Sensory Processing Disorders

Difficulties in the process of choosing, inhibiting, amplifying, integrating, comparing and storing sensory information are known as sensory processing disorders.

Children with sensory processing disorders assimilate certain sensory impressions in the brain differently – weaker, stronger, contorted or not at all – and therefore react for us inappropriately (cf. Becker, Steding-Albrecht 2006).

To date no clear cause of sensory processing disorder has been identified. Possible factors may be negative influences during pregnancy, premature birth, birth injuries, severe infections or serious mental trauma (cf. Becker 2005).

3.2   Assessment of Perception

Further to the motor development screening of the 1.5 to 4 year olds, children with EB aged between 4 and 10 years have been assessed for their tactile, vestibular and proprioceptive perception.

The clinical observation according to Ayres has been used (cf. Becker, Steding-Albrecht 2006; Fisher et al. 1991).

Clinical Observation of Sensory Integration According to Ayres

This is a non-standardised observation instrument to assess the motor abilities of a child. It consists of about 20 tasks; some are verbal requests and some are mimicry of gestures. The following abilities are assessed:

- Prone extension position
- Muscle tone
- The degree of dissociation of the head and trunk as well as the extremities, head – eyes, tongue – lips
- The maturity of the bilateral coordination
- The quality, fluidity and accuracy of movement
- Vestibular and adaptive reactions

- The coordination of motion, postural security and fine motor elements
- Assuming and maintaining postures, motor planning and anticipation (cf. Becker, Steding-Albrecht 2006; Fisher et al. 1991)

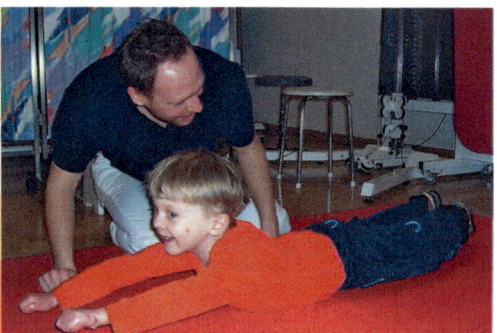

◨ **Fig. 3.1** Prone extension position

3.2.1 Clinical Observation of Children with EB – Considerations

Prior to Starting
- **Meaningfulness of the observation**
  It should be considered that such a clinical observation is only meaningful when the child has already developed the basic motor functions. Especially with DEB this is not always the case.
  Furthermore, before starting the observation the child should be inspected to note the degree of blistering and skin injury. In the case of severe acute blistering on the soles of the feet, knees, abdomen or back it should be considered whether the examination can be performed.
- **Initial interview about the motor development to date**
  In the initial interviews with parents and the examinations of children with EB aged between 1.5 and 4 years it appears that many of these children show delayed motor development. The parental questionnaire focusing on early motor development on p. 18 can be used to discover whether the reasons are EB specific. This information can be very useful for therapists in interpreting the assessment. For example when the child first walked unsupported at 2.5 years, this must be taken into consideration when observing the vestibular reaction at 4 years.

Performing the Assessment
- **Blisters and sores**
  Blistering may have an influence on performance, especially on tasks carried out in the prone position (e. g. prone extension) or on all fours (e. g. tonic neck reflex test). Performance of tasks for the vestibular system (e. g. Schilder's arm-extension test) may also be affected by blisters on the soles of the feet.

Similarly some of the additional items such as standing on one foot or hopping may cause problems. Some relief may be achieved by performing the tasks on a gymnastic mat, but then it must be remembered that the soft supporting surface requires a higher level of vestibular performance than a hard floor. It may be wise to leave out some tasks to prevent blistering and pain. Hopping, for example can put a lot of strain on many children.

- **Contractures**
  When assessing tonic postural or support reactions any contractures and imbalance of muscle function in the knees, hips, trunk and neck must be taken into consideration. The full pronation and supination may be affected by contractures and must be considered when assessing diadochokinesia.
  Checking the slow motions of arms to shoulders and the return to full extension, which is one of the criteria, may be limited by the restricted elbow extension in children with EB.

- **Mutilations and pseudosyndactyly (webbing) of the fingers and toes**
  Children with mutilations, pseudosyndactyly and contractures in the hands as a result of RDEB-HS (recessive DEB Hallopeau-Siemens) have very severe limitations of finger movement (cf. Laimer et al. 2003).
  The testing of the thumb–finger opposition is often impossible.
  Foot deformities and webbing of the toes, especially the big toe, have a large influence on stability while standing or walking and on equilibrium.

- **Eyes**
  There may be complications involving the eyes in children with JEB and DEB. When testing eye movements, following a moving object may be affected by scarring (cf. Laimer et al. 2003).
  Inflammation and hypersensitivity to light may also be present.

- **Oral motor skills**
  Some children with DEB und JEB may have microstomia (small mouth) and adhesions of the tongue and gums (cf. Laimer et al. 2003) so that observation of the tongue and lip movements may be restricted.

- **Ball games**
  For tasks with the ball an inflatable ball should be used to prevent injury.

3.2.2   Useful Additions for Children with EB

The following items may be added to the clinical observation:
- **Standing on one foot**
- **Gait assessment**
- **Climbing wall bars or ladder**
- **Climbing stairs**
- **Motor coordination:** Leaping, spread eagle jumps and jumping jacks may be carried out, but beware of blisters on the soles of the feet.

3

Tactile Perception

Tactile perception is not given much consideration in the clinical observation. Assessment possibilities for this are:

- **Localisation of touch** on the hands: The therapist touches different places on the hand with a light paintbrush. The child has his/her eyes closed and should point to the touched place.

  To achieve standard values the item 'Finger localisation' from the Miller Assessment for Preschoolers (MAP)[1] may be used.

- **Two-point discrimination** on the hands (meaningful from the age of approximately 6–7 years): Using a two-point discrimination tester (see Fig. 3.2) the therapist touches the fingers or palm of the hand while the child has his/her eyes closed. The child should be able to feel this and say whether it is one or two points.

  The standard value on the tip of the index finger is 2–5 mm, whereas on the proximal phalanx it is 6–10 mm (cf. Waldner-Nilsson 2009).

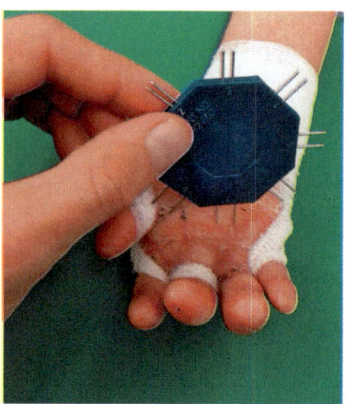

● **Fig. 3.2** Two-point discrimination

- **Texture discrimination** with different surfaces: The child is given small blocks with different surfaces in each hand and, with his/her eyes shut, must say whether the two are the same or different.

- **Stereognosis:** The child feels typical everyday objects in a bag, such as a pencil, marble, spoon or building block, with his/her eyes shut and either names the object or points to the same object on the table. From the age of 5 years, shapes such as a square, triangle, star or moon may be used to take into account the child's increasing abilities. Standardised values from MAP, such as the item 'Stereognosis', may be used. For children aged between 4.0 and 8.11 years the item 'Manual form perception' (MFP) from the Sensory Integration and Praxis Test (SIPT)[2] may be used.

---

1   The MAP tests motor, sensory and cognitive abilities – standardised for children between 2.9 and 5.8 years.
2   The SIPT tests tactile, vestibular and proprioceptive abilities, form and space perception, visuomotor coordination, praxis, bilateral integration and sequencing.

The exact discrimination of surfaces, forms and structure of objects is an ability which requires the coordination of tactile and proprioceptive senses.

3.3   Assessment Results

To date experience and observation show that children with EB have deficits primarily in the vestibular and proprioceptive systems.
This is shown by the following points:

- Poor ability to right the body against the pull of gravity
- Difficulty with the adaptation of muscle tone to the motor task
- Poor posture in sitting and standing
- Deficits in adjusting the right force for the demands of the task and accuracy of movement
- Limited perception of the accurate positioning of head and extremities
- Instability and poor balance in tasks requiring equilibrium
- Problems with timing of coordinated exercises (e. g. catching a ball)
- Deficits in motor coordination

On the whole, these children have a tendency to move slowly and carefully. However, it must be emphasised that this does not apply to all children with EB. Depending on the severity and form of the condition as well as the personality and social environment of the child, many enjoy physical exercise in spite of the pain.

There is no significant deficit of tactile perception even in cases of scarring, webbing or pseudosyndactyly of the hands. No deficit was observed in tactile discrimination or stereognosis, nor was there any tactile defensiveness. In some cases hyperaesthesia in areas of scarring from operations to separate the fingers has been observed, especially when operations had been repeated.

3.3.1   Discussion of the Results

Looking at the effects which EB has on the early motor development (p. 19), it can be assumed that these problems have little to do with any central processing but are caused far more by delays in motor development and lack of experience.

Many children move very little and then very carefully because of the restriction EB puts on them. All movements which cause tension, pressure, friction or resistance are difficult for them because this increases blistering.

Blistering can often limit any equilibrium activities because they must be careful not to fall. Moreover, because the responses from the proprioceptive and vestibular stimuli are partially responsible for the muscle tone, this may be the cause of the lack of tone frequently observed in the general posture.

From what is seen with regard to tactile senses, it appears that if there is any problem this is due to damage to the receptors in the skin (postoperative hyperaesthesia) and not to any central processing.

In conclusion it can be said that knowledge to date indicates the verification of the first hypothesis. This places the cause of the problems on the limited experience due to the condition. The first hypothesis also assumes that there is damage to the peripheral receptors. This cannot yet be verified except for the cases of postoperative hyperaesthesia.

3.4   Occupational Therapy

All the knowledge that has been collected shows that it is important to consider the motor and perceptual development in children with EB. This has been given little attention in the past. Even though there is not much indication of poor tactile perception, this should be included in the assessment if this is to give a holistic picture of the child.

Problems in motor and perceptual functions have a strong influence on the participation and occupational abilities in daily life. Both the social integration (e. g. in the school community) and higher cognitive skills (e. g. learning to read and write, concentration, being attentive or having endurance) may therefore be limited. OT intervention in the areas of motor and perceptual functions can counteract this. Furthermore, the development of contractures and muscle dystrophy can be slowed down by improving posture and by exercise. Being active can strengthen the immune system, which is often weakened by the constant need for wound healing.

3.4.1   Occupational Therapy Intervention Focusing on the Development of Perception

The therapeutic intervention can be orientated to the perceptual disturbances but taking the special needs of children with EB into consideration.

In designing the treatment room the basic rules on p. 24 must be followed carefully. The techniques for minimising injury from pressure and friction described there can also be useful.

Examples of Treatment for the Proprioceptive and Vestibular Systems

The challenge in treating the problems connected with the proprioceptive system is in avoiding pressure and friction. It is necessary to consider what possibilities can be created so that the child receives clear signals from his/her body, experiences the position of his/her head and extremities, and learns to regulate the amount of muscle power needed.

For training the vestibular system slides, hammocks, scooter boards, etc. are used. It is necessary to find ways to minimise pressure and friction. Balancing courses may have the danger of falling and thus injury.

- Using a sheepskin on a slide reduces friction.
- Using a roller slide (see Fig. 3.3) reduces friction. If the child sits in a padded cart there is no friction at all (see Fig. 3.4).
- Special padding (see Fig. 3.5) can be used on scooter boards to reduce pressure on knees, ankles and abdomen.

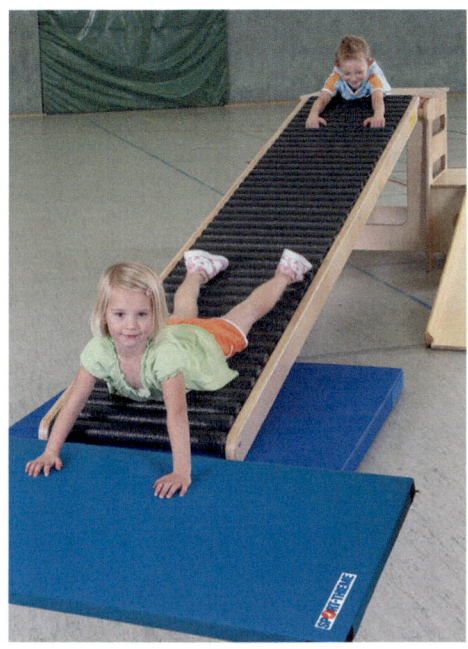

■ **Fig. 3.3** Roller slide (Sport Thieme; www. sport-thieme.com)

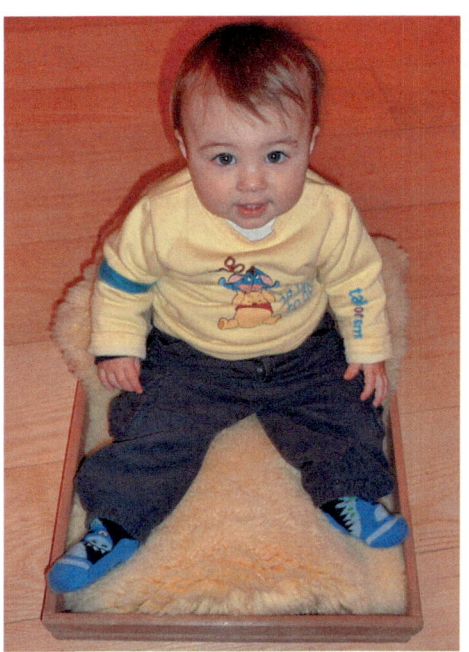

■ **Fig. 3.4** Sheepskin-padded cart for sliding

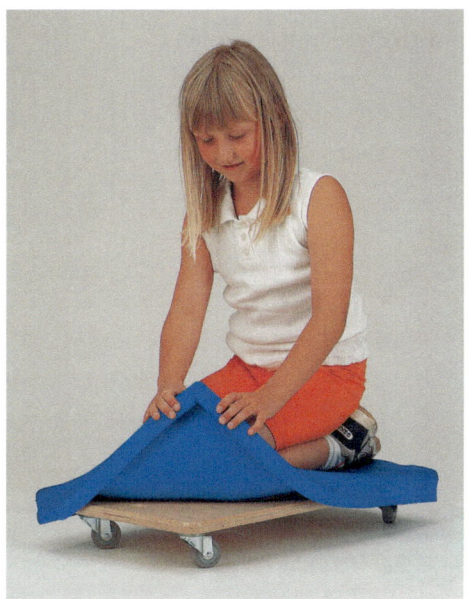

■ **Fig. 3.5** Padding for a scooter board (Sport Thieme; www.sport-thieme.com)

3

- Platform swings are usually padded on the sides. For children with EB it is sensible to use an extra padding on the seat and to wrap the rope with a soft material to give a softer support.
- Hammocks are usually so made that the child is enclosed. In this way, not only vestibular stimuli, but also feedback via the skin as well as proprioception can be experienced. When climbing in and out, friction occurs, so children with EB can use a padded board to prevent this (see Fig. 3.6).

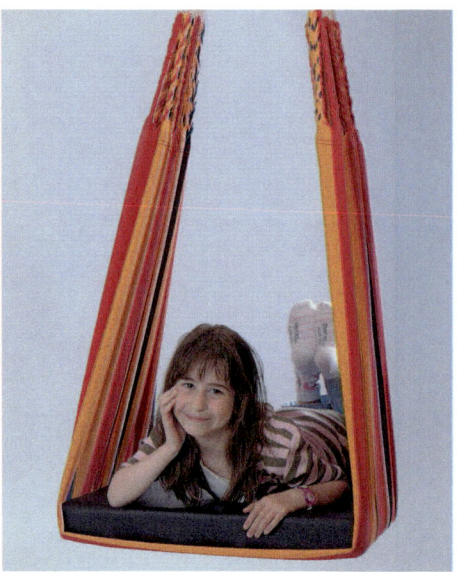

☑ **Fig. 3.6** Padded board for a hammock (Sport Thieme; www.sport-thieme.com)

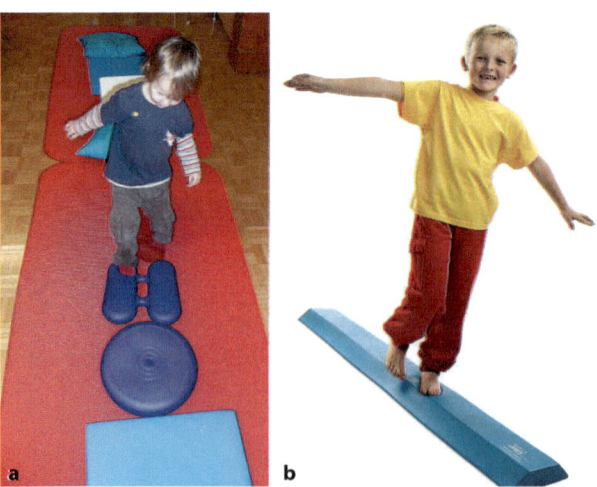

a   b

☑ **Fig. 3.7** Equilibrium training course for children with EB. **a** Balance training course made out of cushions, foam blocks, sand bags and air-cushions. **b** Airex® Balance Beam (Wehrfritz)

- Balancing on floor apparatus lowers the danger of injury but still provides the opportunity to train the equilibrium reactions. Soft gymnastic mats laid underneath provide further padding. Elements of covered foam from a soft play area as pictured on p. 25 can be used to build a balance training course. Sandbags, balance boards, soft mattresses, air cushions or special Airex® balance beams may be used (see Fig. 3.7a,b and Fig. 3.8a–c). The muscles and arches of the feet will also be trained through the use of a balance training course because the foot must constantly adapt to the different surfaces.

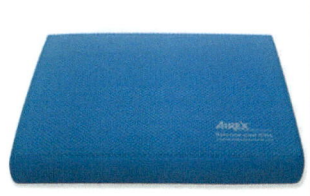 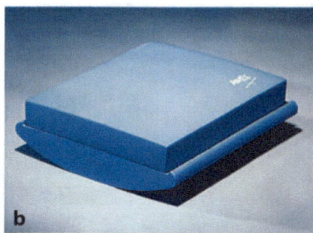 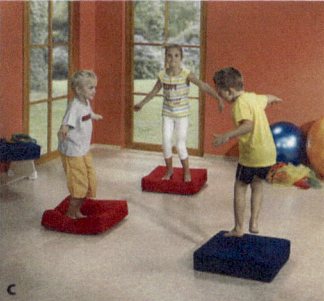

a   b   c

🔲 **Fig. 3.8** Balancing elements for children with EB. **a,b** Airex® Balance-Pad and Airex® Balance-Pad Plus (Sport Thieme; www.sport-thieme.com). **c** Bouncing cushion (Wehrfritz)

- Apart from using adapted wall bars (see p. 26), steps made of foam and covered with soft material can be used to experience heights (see Fig. 3.9).

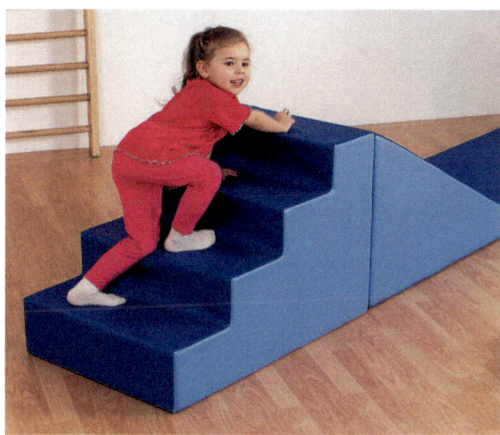

🔲 **Fig. 3.9** Steps made of foam and covered with soft material (Wehrfritz)

- A mini-trampoline (see Fig. 3.10) or a bouncing mattress (see Fig. 3.11) also encourages balancing and motor coordination. The resulting pressure can usually be well accepted.
- Therapy rolls and barrels can be used as well as adapted hammocks and platform swings to encourage righting against the pull of gravity (see Fig. 3.12).

3

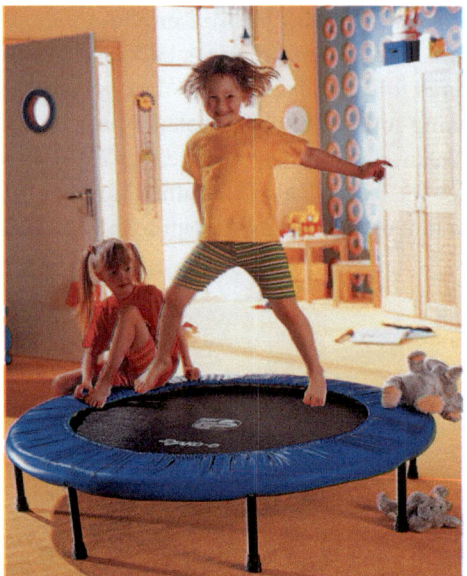

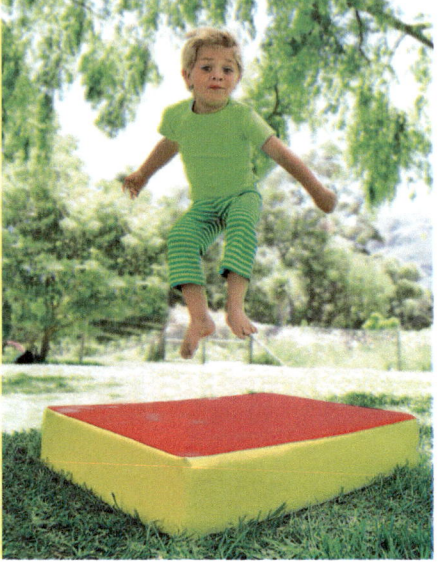

■ **Fig. 3.10** Mini-trampoline (JAKO-O)

■ **Fig. 3.11** Bouncing mattress (Wehrfritz)

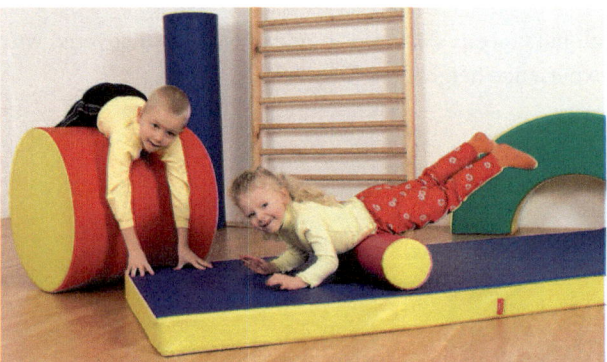

■ **Fig. 3.12** Therapy roll and barrel (Wehrfritz)

- Ropes, which are often used in OT so that a child can pull against his/her own weight, are not usually suitable for children with EB because of the difficulty of holding the rope and the friction it causes.
- Foam elements in the form of a tunnel can be used to creep or crawl through (see Fig. 3.13a,b). The child can train the accurate positioning of his/her head and extremities without serious danger of injury.

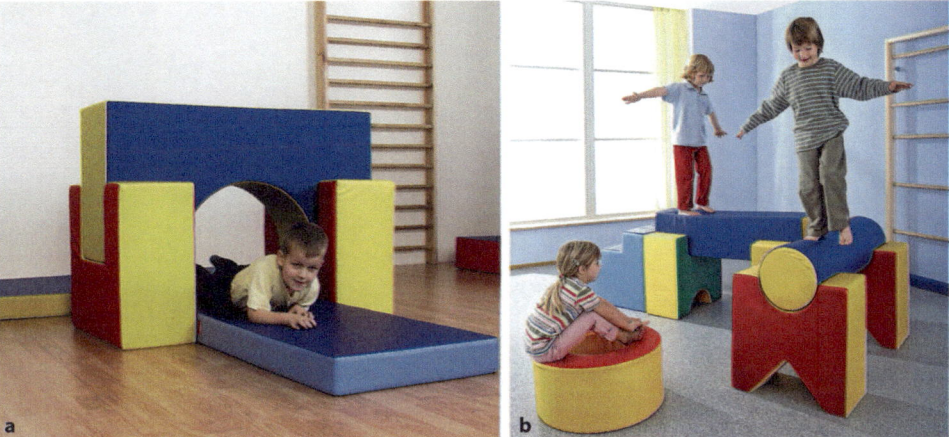

◘ **Fig. 3.13a,b** Foam elements (Wehrfritz)

- Inflatable soft balls, foam balls or soft foam Frisbees can be used to improve the timing or the accuracy in throwing and catching.

Tactile Perception

To improve the tactile sense, the usual therapeutic material such as shaving cream, therapeutic putty, lentil and dried bean baths can be used. In the case of a sand bath, very fine sand is best because of the minimal friction it causes. There may be a danger of infection when open sores on the hands are present.

Parental Counselling

Some of the activities and equipment described above can be used, and extended, by parents at home, who thus integrate them into everyday life.

4 Development of Hand Functions

Florian Prinz

Hands are used to make contact with other people and to accomplish daily tasks and needs. Hands play an important role in professional life and in leisure activities. A faultless prehension influences many areas of everyday life and the participation in various roles. The maturing of prehension begins very early and can be severely restricted by EB. Therefore from the occupational therapist's point of view it is especially important. An outline of the development of prehension is given as background information.

4.1 Development of Prehension (Grasp)

1 Month
The hands of a newborn are usually in slight flexion. Touching the palms of the hands stimulates the grasp reflex, the fingers open and close in an uncoordinated manner.

2–4 Months
Coincidental grasping on tactile stimulation; the infant holds tightly anything that is put into his/her hand and grasps things in the immediate environment. At about 2 months the infant grips with an ulnar palm grip. The grasp development continues radially and the forearm is in pronation.

4–6 Months
Radial palmar grip: The object is fixed against the palm of the hand with all the fingers flexed; the thumb is abducted. The infant plays with his/her hands and fingers, and puts them into his/her mouth. Eye–hand coordination and hand–mouth coordination develop. The infant reaches out towards objects, at first with both hands, then with one. From about 5 months it can also grasp when the arm is in supination. From about 6 months the infant drops objects intentionally.

7–9 Months
The infant becomes more skilled with his/her hands. It passes objects across the midline of the body from one hand to the other and can hold an object in each hand simultaneously.

Lateral pinch grip (key grip) – the infant holds small objects between the pad of the extended thumb and the lateral side of index finger; there is no opposition.

10–12 Months
Pinch grip: The infant grips small objects by opposing the thumb against the index finger. The metacarpophalangeal (MCP) joint of the index finger is flexed and the proximal interphalangeal (PIP) and distal interphalangeal (DIP) joints are extended.

Isolated index finger movements are used to poke into holes and a precision grip develops – a small object is held between the thumb and the index finger with the PIP and DIP joints in flexion and the thumb in opposition.

The pressure can be regulated to some extent.

By the end of the first year, all basic grip functions are developed. In the following years, the toddler becomes more skilled, more accurate and is able to regulate pressure; the fine motor coordination improves.

12–24 Months (Second Year)
Using 'tools': The toddler learns to use a spoon and to hold a drinking cup with both hands. Pencils are used to scribble and a tower of four to six blocks can be built. The toddler can push a button through a slot and place round shapes into a shape-sorting box.

24–36 Months (Third Year)
The child learns to dress him-/herself and to open zips. He/she can turn the pages of a book more easily. The dominance of one hand becomes more obvious. He/she begins to pour water or sand in play without spilling much.

36–48 Months (Fourth Year)
The water tap can be opened. Turning or screwing movements are successful. A glass of water can be carried without spilling. The child begins to use scissors to cut with. He/she builds with Duplo bricks and can open and close larger buttons and zips.
The regulation of pressure is more refined.

Fifth Year
The child can cut along a line smoothly with scissors. Simple shapes like a circle or triangle can be cut out. He/she can put a key into the keyhole and turn it, and can thread small beads. A ball is caught with both hands.

Sixth Year
Tools are used increasingly and with greater skill. Nails can be hit with a hammer and the use of knife and fork is satisfactory but not fully coordinated. It is possible to spread something on bread independently. Small pegs can be skilfully manipulated into a peg-board; shoelaces can be tied.

Seventh Year
The hand development is complete. Tools are used ergonomically, pressure and grip strength are well regulated, and the development of hand dominance is complete (cf. Steding-Albrecht 2003).

4.2   Assessment of Children with EB

To assess the prehension development and fine motor abilities, a play situation suitable for the age is best.

Most important is the recognition of the restrictions caused by deformities and their effect on the occupational abilities of the child in everyday life (play and independence).

Observing the different grips and methods of grasping (e. g. pinch grip, precision grip, opposition and abduction of the thumb) is important with toddlers from the age of 12 months because they may already be restricted, depending on the form of the condition.

Building bricks are very suitable for the observation of bimanual manipulations. Apart from the grasping function, the maturity of the spatial perception as well as the development of play can be assessed when using a shape-sorting box (see Fig. 4.1a,b).

At 18 months a toddler can build a tower with three or more bricks (vertical building); at about 24 months toddlers begin to place bricks beside each other in a row (horizontal building). At about 2.6 years both forms of building are combined and, for example a tunnel for a train can be built (cf. Largo 2007).

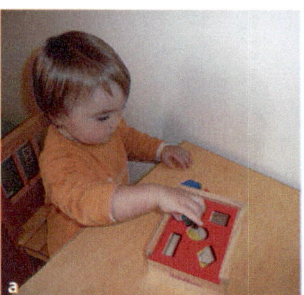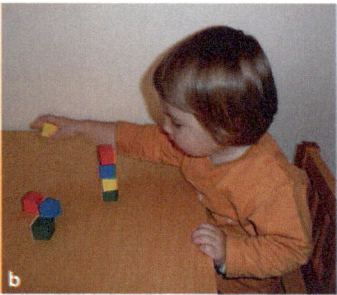

◻ **Fig. 4.1** Playing with building bricks. **a** Placing shapes into a shape sorting box. **b** Building a tower

When manipulating small balls, precision grip, accuracy and eye–hand coordination can be observed (see Fig. 4.2a,b). Two-year-old toddlers should be able to pick up a ball with a spoon.

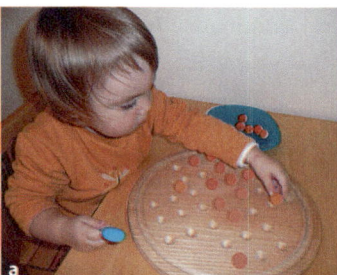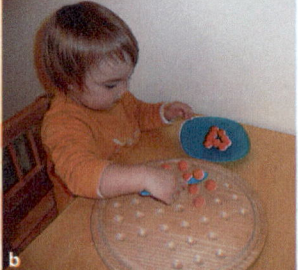

◻ **Fig. 4.2a,b** Manipulating small balls

Simple threading games show accuracy, fine adjustment of grip strength and bimanual coordination (see Fig. 4.3).

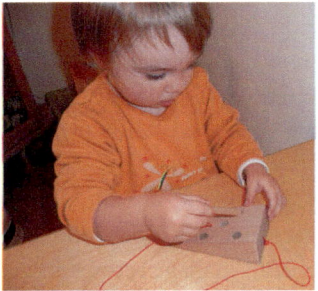

◻ **Fig. 4.3** Toddler manipulates a simple threading game

In the observation of older children (from about 4 years) the emphasis is on the assessment of the use of tools and the maturity in manipulation of complex tasks.

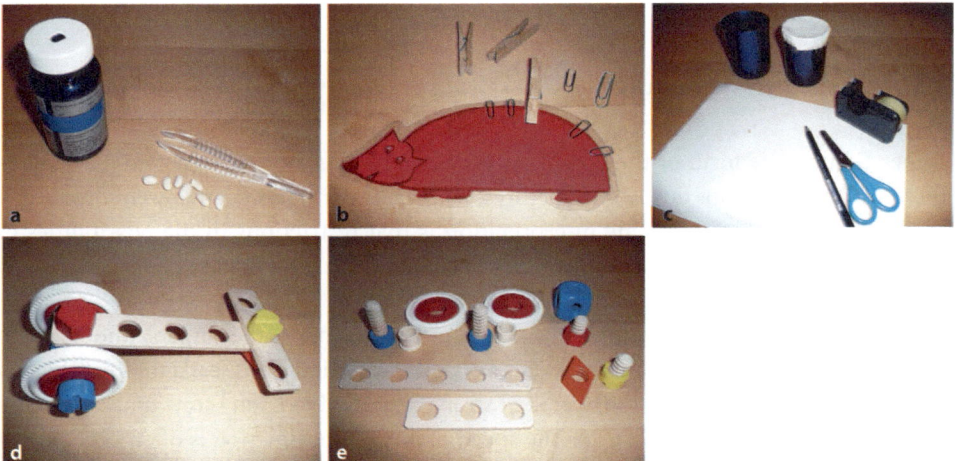

◻ **Fig. 4.4** Assessment suggestions for children from about 4 years. **a** Tweezers game. **b** Hedgehog with clothes pegs and paper clips. **c** Use of pencil, scissors and sticky tape to make a small 'drum'. **d,e** Building a lawn mower with a construction toy, e. g. Baufix

With a simple tweezers game (see Fig. 4.4a), grasping a cylindrical object and opening a screw top, e. g. the little jar pictured, can be assessed. Both of these activities can be difficult for children with EB because of their often-limited abduction of the thumb.

Furthermore, the fine adjustment of pressure, accuracy and eye–hand coordination can be assessed. If dried beans are picked up in one hand, in-hand manipulation can be observed when the beans are moved singly from the handful to a precision grip and then dropped one by one through a small hole into a container.

Clothes pegs or paper clips can be placed on the hedgehog (see Fig. 4.4b), thus showing how skilled the manipulation is and whether there is any restriction or handicap.

Cutting simple shapes (circle, triangle, rectangle – from 5 years) with scissors indicates the use of this tool and any possible handicap can be observed.

In the making of a small 'drum' it is possible to observe how tools relevant to this age (scissors, pencil, sticky tape) are used (see Fig. 4.4c). Apart from this a high degree of praxis ability and spatial perception is required. This task can be achieved by children from the age of about 5 years.

Building a 'lawn mower' with construction toys (e.g. Baufix) requires planning and spatial perception. This is possible from about 5 or 6 years (see Fig. 4.4d,e). A child with deformities of the hand is able to show whether he/she is able to manage screws and to hold cubes or other building shapes.

As the child gets older, independence becomes ever more important to him or her. This is to a large extent dependent on the ability of the child to grasp and hold, and so the subject of independence in everyday life has been given a complete chapter to itself (see p. 59). There further possibilities of activities of daily living (ADL) assessment are given; they overlap partly with what has been described here.

4.3 Assessment Results

Depending on the form of the condition very different results are observed. So long as there are no restrictions due to contractures, mutilations or webbing, many children show a high degree of dexterity. One interpretation is that restrictions in the possibilities of gross motor exploration, which frequently occur, have meant a greater concentration on fine motor activities.

Children with DEB have limited flexion and extension of the fingers, and severely limited thumb mobility, especially abduction and opposition. This leads to difficulties in holding objects, in adjusting the degree of strength needed to open screw tops or picking up small objects in a precision grip. The speed of fine motor function is often very slow.

In spite of the restrictions of grasp in children with DEB, they are usually able to participate in a number of fine motor activities, e.g. building with Lego blocks, cutting out simple shapes with scissors, threading wooden beads and holding flat objects like biscuits. The restriction of finger movement is usually compensated for by holding things between the two deformed hands or a lateral pinch grip, which is often possible.

4.4 Occupational Therapy

The therapeutic intervention for hand function is as individual and as varied as the restrictions or handicaps of the children. Here it is important to note that in severe forms of EB there is often only a very limited range of therapeutic possibilities.

The foremost aim is to enable the child to experience, despite his/her handicaps, as much as possible that typical children experience, and to enable him/her to become and remain as independent as possible in all aspects of daily life.

- In the case of severe hand deformities the aim is to retain functions as long as possible by using anti-webbing techniques or splinting (see p. 123), focusing on compensation mechanisms for grasping and holding or learning trick movements.
- Adaptations and technical devices for the individual needs play a large role in developing independence in daily life. More on this subject is in Chap. 6, 'Independence in Everyday Life and Provision of Assistive Devices' (see p. 59).
- Sometimes compression gloves can further limit hand function. Simple adjustments to the glove, e. g. releasing the IP joint of the thumb, can be extremely useful to the child.

5 Graphomotor Skills

Florian Prinz

Painting, drawing and writing play an important role in the everyday life of children. Writing is especially needed for success in school life and so, as an activity of daily life, it is an important factor in the occupational therapy (OT) intervention. As the typical development plays a part in the assessment of this ability, it is summarised here.

5.1   Development of Pencil Grasp and of Drawing Skills

12–24 Months (Second Year)

The first experiences of using a crayon are usually coincidental and happen around the end of the first year. Experimenting is in the forefront when using crayons, paper and painting materials. The child has fun leaving a mark with the crayon. First disordered scribbles are created and then gradually circular lines develop.

To begin with, the child holds the crayon in a fist (the point of the crayon is on the ulnar side – a palmar supinate grasp). Gradually, the child changes and holds the crayon so that the point is on the radial side. Head, trunk and the entire posture are stable. The movement is from the shoulder and elbow; the wrist and fingers do not yet move independently. As a rule, the crayon is still passed from one hand to the other.

24–36 Months (Third Year)

The hand preference becomes clearer. Gradually, the stabilising hand (to hold the paper) and the writing hand crystallise. The hand and the eye are already well coordinated for short sequences. The movement remains largely from the shoulder and elbow. The first horizontal and vertical lines, spirals, wavy lines and points are drawn.

36–48 Months (Fourth Year)

The eye–hand coordination improves. At first, a digital-pronate grasp with the index finger extended is used, which soon develops into a pincer grip: All five digits or sometimes the thumb, index and middle fingers (static tripod grip) are used to hold the crayon. In this way the wrist is able to move freely and so, along with the increased coordination and visual control, the first closed circle is achieved. In addition, crosses can be drawn.

Fifth Year

The child begins to hold the crayon in the correct dynamic tripod grip using the thumb, index and middle fingers; writing movements come from the finger joints. The preference for one of the hands becomes obvious. When colouring in, the outlines can be better adhered to. The child can draw a line between two points and can copy a rectangle. Pictures of objects are drawn.

Pictures of people consist of three parts (tadpole person). Drawings now cover the whole page, though the individual objects do not have the realistic proportions to one another; rather the size and proportions are governed by their importance.

Five to Seven Year Olds

Towards the end of the fifth year the child begins to draw diagonals. Pictures become more ordered; using, for example a base line, the objects and figures stand on the ground and clouds float in the air. A person is drawn with six parts and simple schematic pictures can be copied. The child can write his/her own name in block capitals as well as single letters, but writing is more a matter of copying forms.

The maturity of the graphomotor skills is so far developed that the child is able to learn to write. Apart from the basic ability accuracy and speed are then also required (cf. Steding-Albrecht 2003; Becker, Steding-Albrecht 2006).

5.2 Assessment of Children with EB

Restrictions as a result of deformities are in the forefront of the assessment of graphomotor skills.

5.2.1 Graphomotorische Testbatterie[1]

This standardised test battery was developed in 1986 by Rudolf. Children aged from 4.6 to 6.11 years can be tested with it, and statements can be made regarding the graphomotor development of the child.

The test battery has seven sub-tests. The individual tests measure the perceptual processes, the visuomotor coordination, the control of movement, the hand–finger dexterity and the ability to use the writing implement on the writing surface.

Which skills are measured by which sub-test are described below (cf. Rudolf 1986).

Labyrinth-Test (LT)	– Hand and finger dexterity – Visuomotor coordination – Anticipation of movement – Assessing hand dominance, if necessary
Task-Test (TT)	– Visuomotor coordination – Form constancy and shape recognition – Measurement of the ability to recognise, differentiate and reproduce figures
Symmetrie-Zeichen-Test (SZT) (symmetry drawing test)	– Measurement of the ability to recognise mirror and symmetrical relationships
Synergie-Schreibversuch (SSV) (synergy writing attempt)	– Form and shape recognition – Reproduction from memory

---

1   This is a German assessment instrument and so the name has not been translated.

Graphesthesia-Test (GT) (graphesthesia test)	– Using a pencil and paper, six geometric symbols must be reproduced in succession – the general perceptive and motor abilities, e.g. judging distances, lengths, angles and crossings, etc. are assessed
Graphomotorik-Test (GMT) (graphomotor test)	– Ability to comprehend letter patterns (graphemes) in their structure and to reproduce them
Form- und Gestalt-Test (FGT) (shape consistency test)	– Ability to abstract and discriminate geometric shapes and to reproduce them

This test is very suitable for children with EB because it assesses only the results and ignores such things as how the writing implement is held. Even children who have severe limitations of hand function and are handicapped in how they hold the implement can be tested with this test battery. It is advisable to use the implements prescribed by the test (medium soft pencil or red felt-tipped pen) and not to use any adaptive devices with EB children. In this way the standardised values are not falsified, and it is possible to observe how the child manages with typical writing implements.

The results of the test battery give information as to the development of the graphomotor skills in spite of the handicaps. It allows some conclusions to be drawn as to how far the child will be able to cope with the graphomotor demands of his/her schooling.

An alternative to the *Graphomotorische Testbatterie* for English speakers could be the *Beery-Buktenica Test* of visual-motor integration together with the *SCRIPT (Scale of Children's Readiness in PrinTing)*.

The *Berry-Buktenica Test*, also known as the *Developmental Test of Visual-Motor Integration (VMI)*, is designed to identify deficits in visual perception, eye–hand coordination and fine motor skills such as handwriting. The test can be administered to children from the age of 2 years up to adulthood. It evaluates the visual–motor integration by providing geometric designs ranging from simple line drawings to more complex figures and asking that the designs be copied (cf. Beery et al. 2010).

The *SCRIPT* test is a letter-form copying research test developed by Weil and Amundson (1994). The child is asked to copy 34 letters by using the Zaner–Bloser manuscript alphabet. For scoring, the original criteria provided by Weil and Amundson or modified versions (e.g. Windsor 1995) can be used (cf. Marr et al. 2001; http://ecrp.uiuc.edu/v3n1/marr.html, 2011).

5.2.2 Observation of Drawing and Writing

To be able to analyse the graphomotor abilities of older children (from 6.11 years), graphomotor exercise sheets may be used.

A second possibility is to ask for a writing sample (e.g. the child copies a short text). While this is being done, the therapist can observe such things as holding the writing implement, the pressure used, how the arm of the writing hand is moved across the desk/table, change of direction of strokes, fluidity of movement, speed, endurance, etc.

5.2.3   The Mann-Zeichen-Test[2]

This test was developed in 1949 by Ziler to assist in the determination of school readiness and the possible necessity of special needs schooling. Later it was also used to measure intelligence. Brosat and Tötemeyer (2007), however, confirm in the revised version of the test that it is not suitable as an intelligence test. Rather it gives information about the development of visual–perceptual processing, especially the visuomotor coordination, the figure-ground differentiation and spatial perception of children.

The task in the test is 'draw a person as well as you can'. To do this the child only has one sheet of paper (DIN A4) and a pencil available.

The individual details of the drawn person are evaluated according to 52 criteria; this includes the in- or exclusion of details, while such things as the aesthetics or proportions are not considered. From the results the *Mannzeichen age* (that is the level of development in drawing a person) can be assessed and compared with the actual age of the child to find out whether this is typical or there is a delay.

As it can be assumed that a child draws a person in the way that it perceives him-/herself, the *Mann-Zeichen-Test* can be seen as an indication of the general development the body scheme and own body perception.

It must be noted that a child should not be assessed exclusively on the *Mann-Zeichen-Test* because it is not possible to draw conclusions about the entire development from one drawing (cf. Brosat, Tötemeyer 2007).

Children with EB have to live with a certain degree of pain from babyhood. They are often restricted in their experience possibilities, in their motor development and in their body awareness, and often have deformities of their hands and feet.

The *Mann-Zeichen-Test* can give information not only about their graphomotor skills along with spatial and visual abilities but also about their body perception (e. g. how are the arms, hands and fingers or legs drawn?).

5.3   Assessment Results

Experience to date shows that writing with a pencil is less of a problem for children with EB than might be expected, considering the frequent massive hand deformities.

As long as there are no contractures, mutilations or webbing to cause handicap, children with EB have not been observed to have any more difficulties with the graphomotor skills than typically developed children.

As a rule, even the pressure of holding the pencil only causes problems with very few children. The danger of blistering is relatively small.

However, the movement of the arm across the table causes friction, which can lead to increased blistering on the forearm and the elbow.

---

2   This is a German test which should not be confused with the draw-a-person test, although it is the drawing of a person.

Well-developed graphomotor skills depend on the fine movements of the PIP and DIP joints of the thumb, and middle and index fingers. Children with JEB are often handicapped or have problems because of the scarring and contractures, which limit the range of motion of these joints (see Fig. 5.1c,d).

The writing movements then come much more from the wrist, elbow and shoulder and so the lack of mobility in the fingers can be well compensated, but the writing process is less economic and more tiring. Even so, the speed usually suffices to complete the school requirements (writing in class for short periods).

However, during long periods of writing children with EB become tired more quickly because of the poor economy of effort.

Children with DEB have not only the lack of finger movements, but also can have mutilations, pseudosyndactyly and contractures of the fingers. In some cases their hands have the appearance of mittens which are surrounded by an epidermal cocoon; usually only the thumb is free to move. Such children grasp the pencil, as shown in Fig. 5.1b, with a lateral grip.

If the abduction and opposition of the thumb is severely limited because of adhesions, only very thin pencils can be held.

Through using a lateral grip the hand is held fully in pronation while writing and cannot slide across the paper on the ulnar side as usual. This larger surface causes more resistance and friction, which makes writing even less economic than described above. This means that writing is usually slower and the child tires even more quickly.

Hand dominance: No difference has been observed in hand dominance between children with EB and other children. Further, the dominant hand is no more affected by webbing and contractures than the non-dominant hand (cf. Mullett 1998).

Development of drawing: The majority of the children who have been assessed show a development of drawing compatible with their age, even in cases of severe limitations of pencil grasp (*Mannzeichen age* – see Chap. 5.2.3).

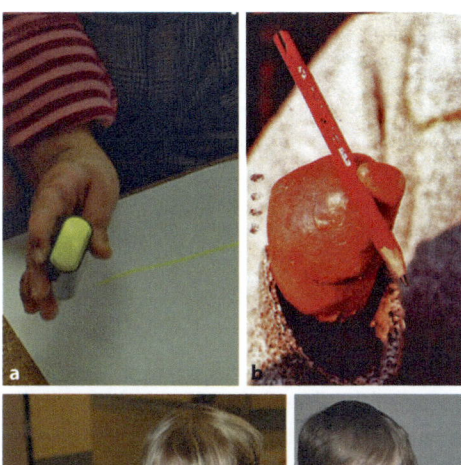
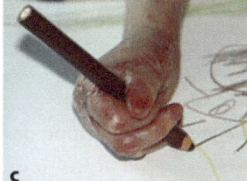
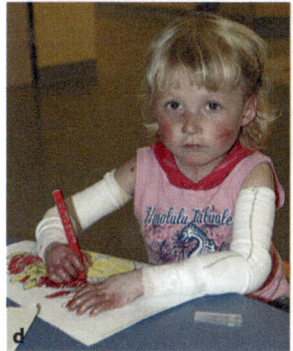
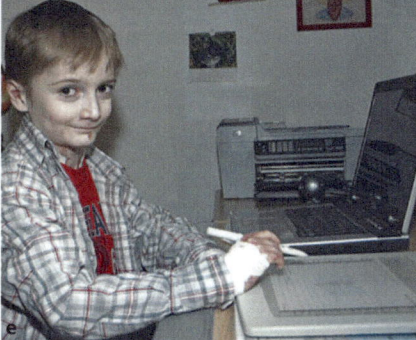

Fig. 5.1 Different ways of holding a pencil in children with EB. **a** Palmar supinate grasp. **b** Lateral grip in the case of an epidermal cocoon (DEBRA Austria). **c–e** Limitations of the finger movements due to scarring and contractures (Hametner)

5.4 Occupational Therapy

The graphomotor problems children with EB have are mostly due to the physical situation of the hands and fingers caused by the condition. OT therefore concentrates on retaining the movement of the wrist and fingers for as long as possible, adapting the pen or pencil to the needs of the child and developing the most economic compensation strategies. It does not aim to improve dexterity or perception.

5.4.1 Occupational Therapy Intervention Focusing on Drawing and Graphomotor Skills

- Most children manage to use customary writing implements quite well. In some cases the use of an ergonomic grip is an improvement, assuming that there is an adequate abduction of the thumb. Figures 5.2a,b show a soft rubber grip which can be used to minimise the pressure while writing. Most other available assistive writing devices (e. g. triangular ones) have been shown to be less satisfactory because they are made of a hard material and have sharp corners.

5

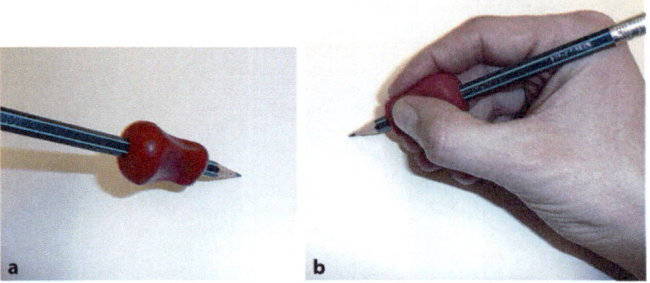

🔲 Fig. 5.2a,b Pencil grip – ergonomic writing device

- For children who have a very limited abduction of the thumb (see Fig. 5.1b), an individual grip can easily be made by using silicone elastomer (see Fig. 5.3). This reduces the pressure of the side of the pencil on the skin. Because the volume of the pencil is only marginally increased, this variation is suitable for many children with epidermal cocoon deformities of the hand and limited abduction of the thumb.

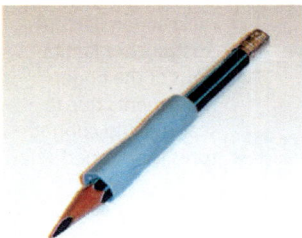

🔲 Fig. 5.3 Pencil thickening made of silicone elastomer

- Clothing made of easy sliding material, e. g. silk, can help the movement of the arm across the table when writing and so minimise the friction. It is also possible to attach sheepskin to the sleeves to ease movement.
- Gel roller pens (see Fig. 5.4) can be used because the roller creates little resistance and so facilitates writing.

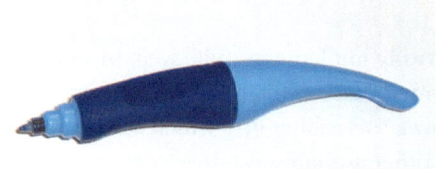

🔲 Fig. 5.4 Ergonomically formed pen with a gel roller system

- If compression gloves are worn, it is important to take care that they do not hinder the child in holding the pencil, e. g. the opposition of the thumb.

Computer Adaptation

- When the hands are very severely handicapped, writing with a pen or pencil can be very tiring so that the use of a computer should be considered. For many children a touch pad or small computer mouse is adequate for good handling (see Fig. 5.5).

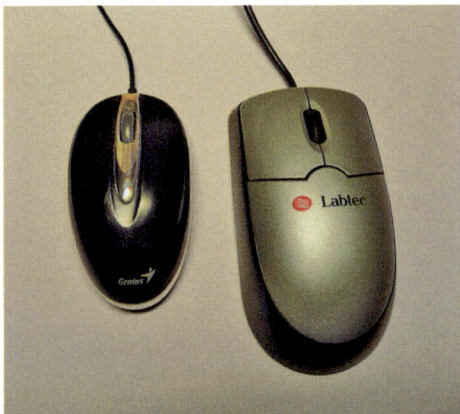

◘ **Fig. 5.5** Small laptop mouse *left* in the picture

- Individual solutions for the handling of a computer can be worked out together with firms which specialise in providing computer adaptations, e. g. using:
  - A mouse that reacts to minimal touch or can be controlled by the thumb alone (see Fig. 5.6a–c)
  - Touch screen
  - Speech-recognition programmes

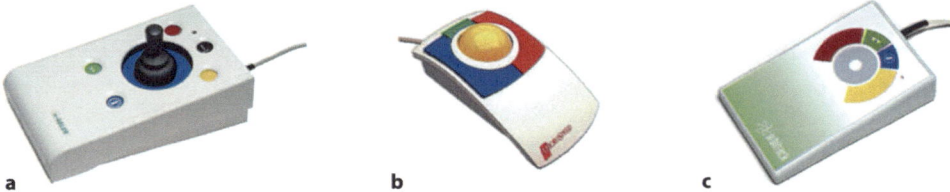

a   b   c

◘ **Fig. 5.6** Assistive devices for the computer. **a** Special PC mouse 'nAbler Joystick' (LifeTool) reacts to minimal touch. **b** Special PC mouse 'Kidtrack Trackball Colour' (LifeTool) with large mouse keys for right- or left-handed people. **c** Special PC mouse 'nAbler Orbitrack' (LifeTool) for children and people with very limited motor abilities

- If neither writing nor typing on the computer is satisfactory, it may be possible to copy some things from fellow pupils, or a dictating machine can be used.

6 Independence in Everyday Life and Provision of Assistive Devices

Hedwig Weiß and Florian Prinz

The assessment possibilities described here present more information and additions to those outlined in Chap. 4, 'Development of Hand Functions', and refer in particular to everyday activities.

6.1 Assessment of Children with EB

Use simple soft items such as bananas to find out how well a child can cut and pick up food with a fork and a spoon. Alternatively, therapeutic putty may be used (see Fig. 6.1a–c).

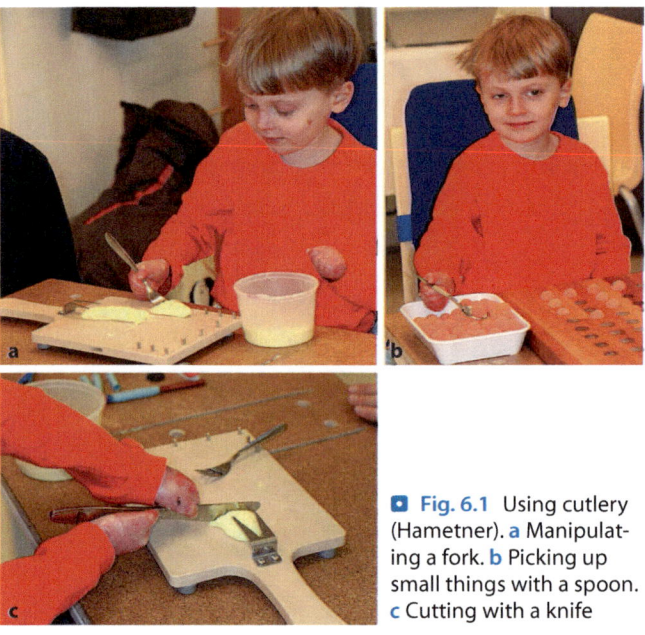

◘ **Fig. 6.1** Using cutlery (Hametner). **a** Manipulating a fork. **b** Picking up small things with a spoon. **c** Cutting with a knife

A board with various fastenings is useful for analysing manipulation problems (see Fig. 6.2). In this way some simple adaptations such as rings on zips can be tried out.

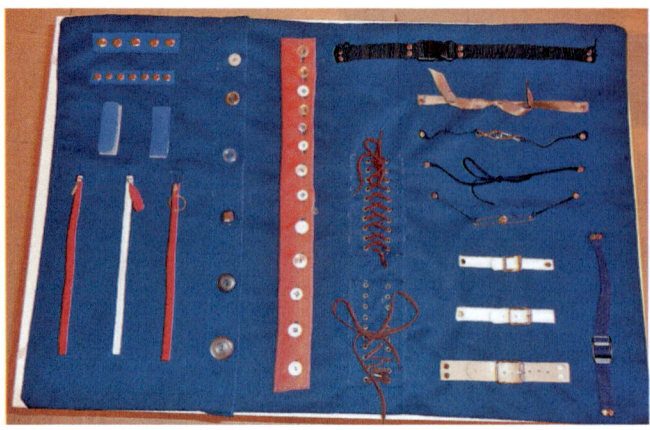

◘ **Fig. 6.2** Fastenings board for the assessment of the manipulation of fastenings

Putting on and taking off clothing and shoes can be done in the assessment situation so as to analyse the difficulties.

Also handling everyday objects can be observed; for example taking coins and bank notes out of a closed purse or wallet (see Fig. 6.3).

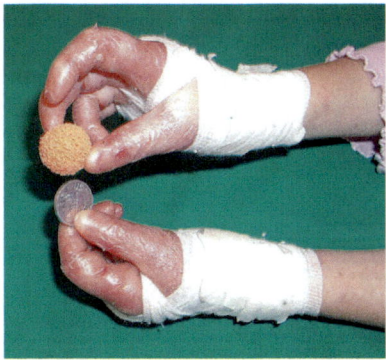

◘ **Fig. 6.3** Handling everyday objects such as coins

Some areas of grooming such as applying cream, combing the hair or cleaning teeth can also be tried out and analysed.

As changing bandages and dressings plays a large role in the life of these clients, it is important to observe this to see whether the client is able to do his or her own bandaging. Children from about 8 or 9 years can be shown how they can help with this as long as they have an adequate hand function (see Fig. 6.4a,b).

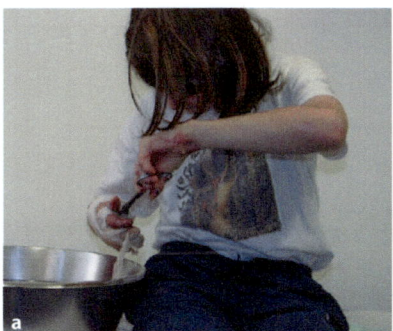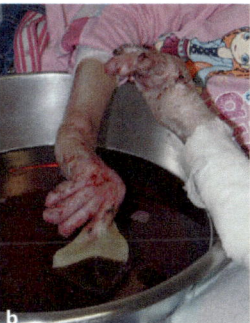

◘ **Fig. 6.4a,b** Independent changing of bandages (Hametner)

The use of electronic devices such as mobile telephones, and MP3 or DVD players can be tried out in therapy.

So as to obtain a comprehensive picture of the abilities and difficulties in everyday life of the client, the parents of the child can be asked to fill out the following questionnaire. Later this can provide valuable details for use in intervention.

6.1.1 Parental Questionnaire Focusing on the Coping Skills of Children with EB in Everyday Life

Parental questionnaire focusing on the coping skills of children with EB in everyday life

Name of child: **Date of birth:**   **Age:**
EB type: **Date:**

Key

☺☺   ☺☺   ☺☺   ☹☹   ✋

very well   well   poor   not at all   with help

Please mark where appropriate   _____

                                                              The line beside the Smileys gives
                                                              space for remarks or additions

---

SELF-CARE

Dressing and undressing

Putting on and taking off underclothes

☺☺   ☺☺   ☺☺   ☹☹   ✋   _____

Putting on and taking off socks/stockings

☺☺   ☺☺   ☺☺   ☹☹   ✋   _____

Trousers

☺☺   ☺☺   ☺☺   ☹☹   ✋   _____

Pullover/T-Shirt

☺☺   ☺☺   ☺☺   ☹☹   ✋   _____

Shirt/jacket

☺☺   ☺☺   ☺☺   ☹☹   ✋   _____

Which types of material are tolerated best?

Cotton ☐   silk ☐   synthetic materials ☐

Other   _____

Putting on and taking off shoes

Outdoor shoes

☺☺   ☺☹   ☹☹   ☹☹   ✋   _____

Does your child use:
Special shoes ☐   inserts ☐   padding ☐

Other _____

Fastenings

Buttons

☺☺   ☺☹   ☹☹   ☹☹   ✋   _____

Shoelaces

☺☺   ☺☹   ☹☹   ☹☹   ✋   _____

Zip

☺☺   ☺☹   ☹☹   ☹☹   ✋   _____

Velcro

☺☺   ☺☹   ☹☹   ☹☹   ✋   _____

Does your child use any adaptive devices or adaptations to make using fastenings easier?

_____

Eating and drinking

Cutting food

☺☺   ☺☹   ☹☹   ☹☹   ✋   _____

Eating with a spoon or fork

☺☺   ☺☹   ☹☹   ☹☹   ✋   _____

Does your child use:
Special cutlery ☐   teaspoon ☐

Other _____

Drinking out of a glass or cup

☺☺   ☺☹   ☹☹   ☹☹   ✋   _____

Hygiene and grooming

Shower

☺☺   ☺☺   ☺☹   ☹☹   ✋   _____

Bath

☺☺   ☺☺   ☺☹   ☹☹   ✋   _____

Does your child use:

Bath board ☐   anti-slip mat ☐

Other _____

Cleaning teeth

☺☺   ☺☺   ☺☹   ☹☹   ✋   _____

Does your child use:

Manual toothbrush ☐   electric toothbrush ☐   special toothbrush ☐

Other _____

Combing/brushing hair

☺☺   ☺☺   ☺☹   ☹☹   ✋   _____

Applying cream

☺☺   ☺☺   ☺☹   ☹☹   ✋   _____

Toileting (including wiping intimate parts)

☺☺   ☺☺   ☺☹   ☹☹   ✋   _____

Sleeping

Mattress/pillow/special protection

Foam mattress ☐   sprung mattress ☐   latex mattress ☐
Water bed ☐   feather pillow ☐   foam pillow ☐
Ergonomic pillow ☐   support cushion(s) ☐   sheepskin protection ☐

Other _____

Material of the bedclothes

Silk ☐   cotton ☐

Other _____

Sleeping position

Back ☐   side ☐   front ☐

Household activities

Opening a bottle

☺☺   ☺☺   ☺☺   ☺☺   ✋   _____

Opening a tin/can

☺☺   ☺☺   ☺☺   ☺☺   ✋   _____

Opening packaging

☺☺   ☺☺   ☺☺   ☺☺   ✋   _____

Preparing a snack

☺☺   ☺☺   ☺☺   ☺☺   ✋   _____

Opening and closing a drawer

☺☺   ☺☺   ☺☺   ☺☺   ✋   _____

Putting an electric plug into a socket and taking it out

☺☺   ☺☺   ☺☺   ☺☺   ✋   _____

Opening and closing a water tap

☺☺   ☺☺   ☺☺   ☺☺   ✋   _____

Shopping

Taking items off the shelf

☺☺   ☺☺   ☺☺   ☺☺   ✋   _____

Taking out coins

☺☺   ☺☺   ☺☺   ☺☺   ✋   _____

Carrying bags

☺☺   ☺☺   ☺☺   ☺☺   ✋   _____

Open the door with a key

☺☺   ☺☺   ☺☺   ☺☺   ✋   _____

LEISURE/HOBBIES

What hobbies does your child have?

Sport ☐ music ☐ drawing/painting ☐ handicraft ☐
Reading ☐ friends ☐ singing ☐

Other _____

Which kinds of sport does your child do?

Horse riding ☐ cycling ☐ swimming ☐ ball games ☐

Other _____

What measures to you take to prevent blistering in sport?

Knee pads ☐ elbow pads ☐ gloves ☐ gel inserts ☐

Other _____

Is your child integrated into a group of friends?

☺☺ ☺☹ ☹☹ ☹☹ _____

Does your child take part in any club or group activities?

Which ones? _____

What relaxation/pain reduction method(s) does your child use?

Relaxation techniques ☐ breathing techniques ☐ massage ☐
Music ☐ sound bed ☐

Other _____

Can you go on holiday with your child?

☺☺ ☺☹ ☹☹ ☹☹ _____

Where do you go and what kind of holiday is best?

Pony club (riding) ☐ city trip ☐

Other _____

What conditions do you and your child need when on holiday?

Bathtub ☐ washing machine ☐ pureed food ☐ air conditioning ☐

Other _____

SCHOOL

Writing with pen/pencil

☺☺   ☺☹   ☹☹   ☹☹   _____

Does your child use a special pen/pencil?

_____

Writing on a PC

☺☺   ☺☹   ☹☹   ☹☹   _____

Does your child use any special adaptations?

Special mouse ☐   touch screen ☐   special keyboard ☐

Other   _____

Speed of writing

☺☺   ☺☹   ☹☹   ☹☹   _____

Is the speed adequate for:

Copying from the board ☐   dictation ☐   tests ☐

Other   _____

Turning pages of a book/magazine/newspaper

☺☺   ☺☹   ☹☹   ☹☹   _____

Using a mobile telephone

☺☺   ☺☹   ☹☹   ☹☹   _____

Using scissors

☺☺   ☺☹   ☹☹   ☹☹   ✋   _____

Does your child use special scissors?

Standard scissors ☐   child's scissors ☐

Loop/self-opening scissors ☐   table-top scissors ☐

Other   _____

How does your child sit best in the classroom?

At the front ☐   at the back ☐   single place ☐   wheelchair ☐   upholstered chair ☐

Other _____

Does your child have any special device for sitting for long periods?

Padding ☐   rounded seat edge on upholstered chair ☐
Rounded edge of table ☐   rounded corners ☐

Other _____

Carrying a school bag

☺☺   ☺☺   ☺☹   ☹☹   ✋   _____

Does your child use assistive devices or techniques?
One set of books at school and one at home ☐   trolley ☐

Other _____

Does your child have his/her own carer in the school?

For how many hours a day and with what conditions?

_____

What is the best place for your child to spend the breaks in?

In the classroom ☐   in the passage/corridor ☐   in the playground ☐

Is your child integrated into class life?

☺☺   ☺☺   ☺☹   ☹☹   _____

Does your child participate in gymnastics?

☺☺   ☺☺   ☺☹   ☹☹   ✋   _____

Alternatives? _____

Does your child participate in handicraft lessons?

☺☺   ☺☺   ☺☹   ☹☹   ✋   _____

What activities are possible? _____

Is it planned for your child to stay at school beyond the minimum age?

If so with what plans?

_____

What professional opportunities do you see for your child?

_____

MOBILITY

Transfer

Get into bed and get up again

☺☺   ☺☺   ☹☹   ☹☹   ✋   _____

Turnover in bed

☺☺   ☺☺   ☹☹   ☹☹   ✋   _____

Sit down on a chair and get up

☺☺   ☺☺   ☹☹   ☹☹   ✋   _____

Sit down at the table and get up

☺☺   ☺☺   ☹☹   ☹☹   ✋   _____

Sit down on a sofa or armchair and get up

☺☺   ☺☺   ☹☹   ☹☹   ✋   _____

Pick something up from the floor

☺☺   ☺☺   ☹☹   ☹☹   ✋   _____

Get in and out of public transport

☺☺   ☺☺   ☹☹   ☹☹   ✋   _____

Locomotion

Walk

☺☺   ☺☺   ☹☹   ☹☹   ✋   _____

How far?

_____

Run

☺☺   ☺☺   ☹☹   ☹☹   _____

How far?

_____

Go up and down stairs

☺☺   ☺☺   ☹☹   ☹☹   ✋   _____

Cross the street within the time span of the green light

☺☺   ☺☺   ☹☹   ☹☹   ✋   _____

Tricycle

☺☺   ☺☺   ☺☺   ☹☹   ✋ _____

Scooter

☺☺   ☺☺   ☺☺   ☹☹   ✋ _____

Does your child use any special adaptations?
Safety scooter ☐   special handlebars ☐

Other _____

Balance bike

☺☺   ☺☺   ☺☺   ☹☹   ✋ _____

Bicycle

☺☺   ☺☺   ☺☺   ☹☹   ✋ _____

Does your child use any special adaptations?
Balancing wheels ☐   special handlebars ☐   backpedal brake ☐   gel saddle ☐

Other _____

Do you use a wheelchair?

Yes ☐   no ☐

Do you use any special adaptations?
Electric wheelchair ☐   special cushion ☐

Other _____

How does your child go to school?

Private car ☐   school bus ☐   public transport ☐   bicycle ☐   on foot ☐

Other _____

Taking your child in the car

Do you use any special adaptations?
Child safety seat ☐   padded seatbelt ☐   air conditioning ☐

Other _____

6.2   Occupational Therapy Intervention Focusing on Everyday Life and Use of Assistive Devices

6.2.1   Self-Care

Dressing, Undressing

To be able to dress and undress is an important step towards independence in the life of a child. There is a danger, because of the difficulties of grasping and holding things, of doing these tasks for the child when this is no longer necessary.

The process can be simplified if certain rules are followed. On the one hand, the choice of clothing has to be made to prevent friction and pressure, on the other hand, there are adaptations to fastenings, etc. which make it easier to open and close garments.

When choosing garments consider the following:
- No rough labels, lumpy seams or tight elastic
- Wide neckline
- Sportswear is usually breathable and prevents sweating that leads to increased blistering (underclothes, T-shirts, jackets).
- Overalls have no tight waist; trousers with a knitted waistband cause less friction.

TIPS

✓ Prophylactic bandaging can protect against rough seams and fastenings.
✓ Underclothes can be worn inside out so that the seams are on the outside and there is less friction.
✓ To enable an easier way to pull up trousers and underpants loops can be sewn onto the sides.
✓ Use elastic instead of a cuff or buttons on the sleeves of shirts.

Fabrics well tolerated
- Cotton and silk are best
- Synthetic fabrics
- Blended fabrics that stretch (soft and they 'give')
- DermaSilk® from the company Alpretec, a line of therapeutic clothing conceived for people who suffer from skin diseases (http://www.dermasilk.com/)

CAUTION

✓ Too much elastane causes the garment to stick to the body!

Fastenings

- Zips can have a ring or loop added (see Fig. 6.5). To provide an adequate tension on the zip when closing it, a loop can be added at the base of the zip or garment. To make dressing and undressing generally easier, sometimes it is better not to open the zip completely!
- Use large buttons.
- Velcro – possibly add a loop if the Velcro closes exactly (see Fig. 6.6).

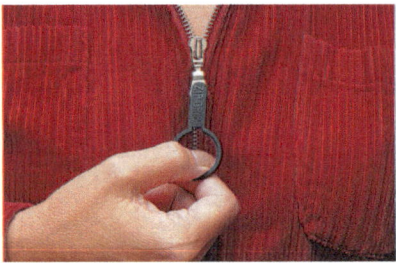

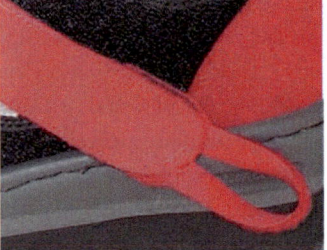

■ **Fig. 6.5** Zip opener (North Coast Medical)   ■ **Fig. 6.6** Velcro adaptation

Socks

- Smooth elastic material
- Socks with no elasticised top

Shoes

Buying shoes for children is a very special subject because they do not feel exactly whether the shoes fit well. The nervous system of children is not well developed enough for them to be aware of pressure points. For this reason, children sometimes put their shoes on the wrong feet and do not notice it.

If you try to feel whether the toes are too tight, the child often pulls the toe back and it is not really possible to tell whether the shoe fits or not.

It is best to measure the feet accurately with special foot-measuring devices which some shoe shops have available. The length and width of the foot can be measured accurately and the shoes selected accordingly. It might be useful to buy such a measuring device to use at home.

> **TIP**
>
> ✓ www.kidsfeet.info gives information and downloads about children's shoes and measuring feet.

It is possible to make a cardboard pattern by drawing round the foot onto a piece of cardboard, cutting it out and then placing this in the shoe to see how well it fits. The shoe should be about 1.2 cm longer because the foot slides forward in the shoe while walking.

The sole of the shoe should be flexible in all directions; only then does it allow for the correct foot movement: rolling from heel to toe. Rubber soles offer a good shock absorption; leather ones are too thin.

The material should be soft and breathable and the sole non-slip. Däumling, Superfit, GEOX, Elefanten, etc. are good makes of children's shoes. Velcro is easier to handle than shoelaces. It is also possible to add on a small tab to make the opening of it easier.

When deciding on the width of the shoe, it is important to remember that it must be possible to insert the thumb at the instep, and with EB children, of course bandaging must be considered.

There are a number of inserts for foot correction, e. g. flatfoot. Such inserts are a passive measure and do not replace training of the foot muscles. Sheepskin or gel inserts may be tried to reduce pressure on the foot (see Fig. 6.7).

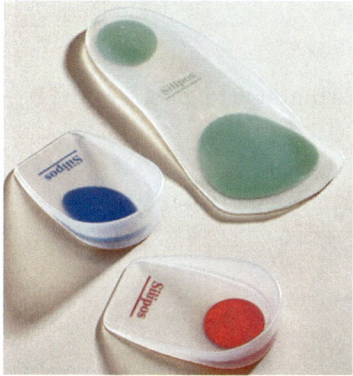

🔲 **Fig. 6.7** Gel inserts to prevent blistering (North Coast Medical)

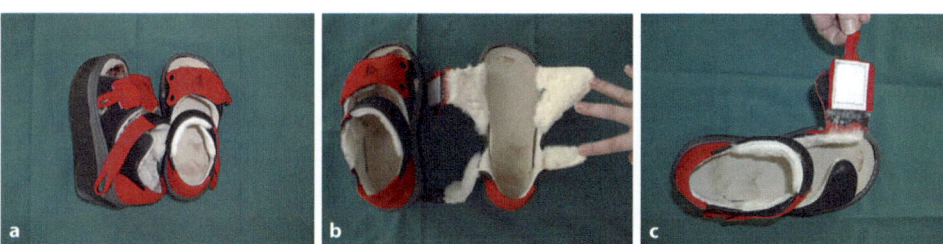

🔲 **Fig. 6.8a–c** Medical shoes with sheepskin padding and Velcro fastening adaptation

If the shoes are second-hand the sole needs to be checked in case it has worn unevenly.

The shoe size of a child between 1 and 3 years needs to be checked every 2 months, for a child between 3 and 4 years, every 4 months; and for a child between 4 and 6 years, every 6 months. If there are severe deformities of the feet, and if the skin is extremely sensitive, it pays to have the shoes made by an orthopaedic shoemaker. They can pad vulnerable areas and possibly alter the sole appropriately.

Another possibility are medical shoes (see Fig. 6.8a–c), or diabetic shoes, which are obtainable in various designs, though not very small sizes.

These shoes can be adapted so that the child can open them independently.

Eating and Drinking

Eating and drinking is a subject which may present many and varied problems. On the one hand, a special diet is sometimes necessary to supply an adequately high intake of proteins. On the other hand, some foods cannot be consumed because of their consistency. Apart from that, the usual mealtimes may be insufficient because eating and drinking can take a very long time.

The complications of EB mean that often cutlery cannot be held very easily. It can be too large and too heavy, and there may be insufficient strength to cut up the food.

TIPS

✓ The following links offer information about suitable nutrition for people with EB:
  www.debra-international.org
  www.ebinfoworld.com
✓ To help distract from the pain and effort while eating, children may be allowed to watch television or play computer games.

Eating
- Use children's and/or plastic cutlery
- Cake fork and spoon if normal cutlery is too heavy or cannot be held
- Extra sharp serrated knife for cutting
- Adaptations following bilateral hand surgeries (see Fig. 6.9)

Drinking
- Drinking straws
- Cup with two handles

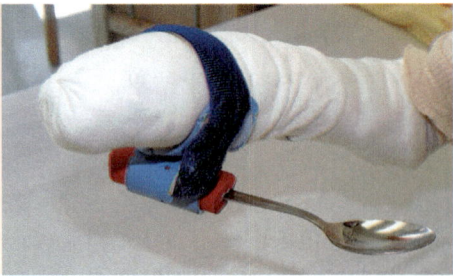

◨ **Fig. 6.9** Adaptation for eating

Bathing and Grooming
Bathroom
The bathroom is a very important room because that is where a lot of time is spent on bandaging and hygiene.

The following measures will make the work there easier:

Bathroom furnishings
- Barrier-free, with wheelchair access (see p. 91)
- Knee space under the wash basin for use with a wheelchair
- Height-adjustable changing table (see Figs. 6.10 and 6.11)
- Roll-in shower without a step for use with a wheelchair
- Surfaces for easy disinfection
- Plenty of space for storage of dressing and bandaging material, towels and linen
- Mirrors to examine all parts of the body
- Moveable lighting
- Door and cabinet handles that can be opened easily independently by people with EB
- Bath seats and boards
- Hot water thermostat, to prevent burning and scalding
- Single lever tap that can be opened with a fist

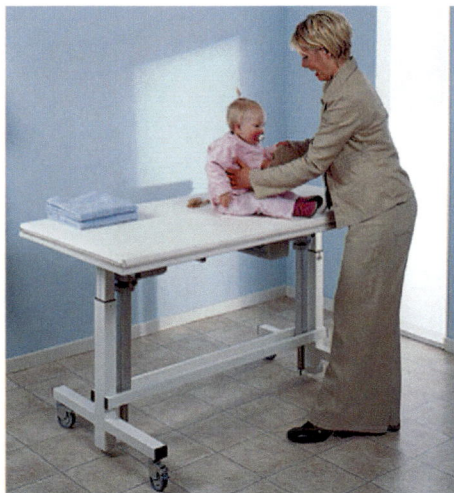
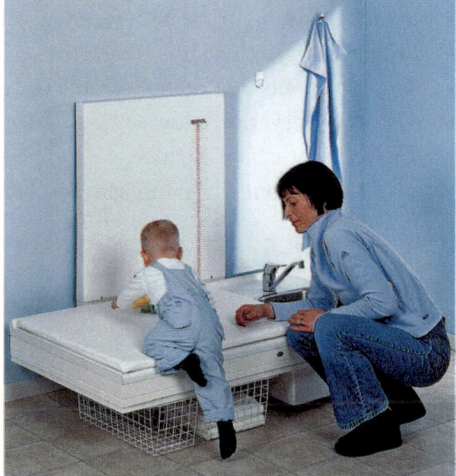

◨ **Fig. 6.10** *Mobilio* – freestanding, mobile and electrically height-adjustable changing table (Matzka Rehatechnik). Freestanding mobile changing table with brakes. The table is stable, fixed but easily adjusted and moved. The height can be adjusted electrically; there is a 3-m-long cable. The adjustment is infinitely variable between 65 and 100 cm with a switch on a spiral cable

◨ **Fig. 6.11** *Maxi* – wall-mounted, height-adjustable changing table with wash basin (Matzka Rehatechnik). Wall-mounted changing table with or without wash basin. Two wire baskets are mounted below the surface. Maxi is mounted on a wall bracket; the height is infinitely variable between 30 and 100 cm with a switch on a spiral cable. The changing table with the wash basin has a cover, a mixer tap with protection against scalding, flexible inlet and outlet pipes with an odour closure device

Mouth Hygiene

Cleaning teeth with either a conventional toothbrush or an electric toothbrush is almost impossible for children who have difficulties opening their mouths (because of microstomia).

Alternatives are:
- Extra-soft toothbrush with short bristles
- Oral irrigator
- Cotton-wool buds
- Mouthwash

Showering
- Shower chair or stool
- Steam shower
- Shower head with very fine soft jet

Bathing
- Place a soft towel in the bathtub to sit on.
- Non-slip mat should be placed.
- If necessary use a bath seat or board (see Fig. 6.12).
- Soak bandaging in the bath (see Fig. 6.13).
- Soften scabs in the bath.
- Use soft towels that do not scratch or rub (dryer).
- Use a hair dryer on a low setting to dry off.
- Use antiseptic bath essence.
- Lift the child out of the tub with one hand under the buttocks, not under the shoulders.

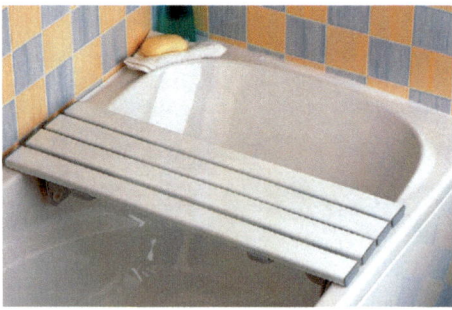

□ **Fig. 6.12** Bath board (Medictools)

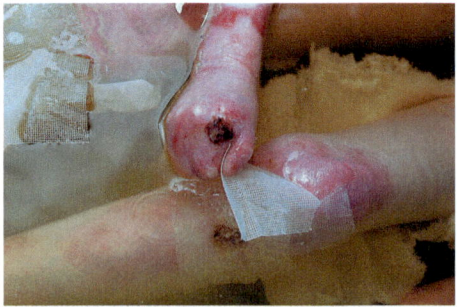

□ **Fig. 6.13** Child soaking and removing bandages in the bath (Hametner)

Toilet
- Barrier-free with wheelchair access
- Wet toilet wipes
- Toilet with bidet and warm air dryer

Sleeping

Experience shows that persons with EB sleep in a wide variety of positions. Lying on the front can place great strain on the cervical spine; using a long pillow placed the length of the body (a body pillow or bolster) can reduce this strain.

Using an ergonomic pillow can also be useful for those who sleep on their side. It is recommended to try out a pillow for a few nights to see if it is really the most suitable one (see Fig. 6.14).

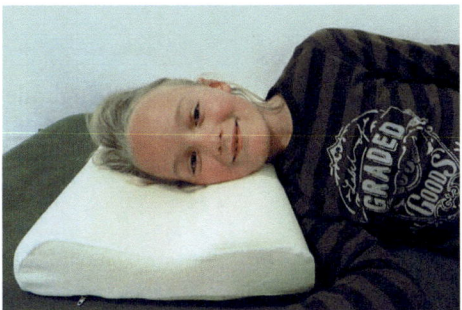

■ Fig. 6.14 Ergonomic pillow

Bedroom furnishing

- Barrier-free and with wheelchair access
- Plenty of storage space for frequent changes of clothes
- Soft padding on the edge of the bed
- Bed without a bed frame
- Large bed
- Fan
- Shade – awning or blind if required

Mattress

A soft mattress made of latex, cold foam or viscoelastic material which adjusts to the shape of the body is the most suitable. Air-filled, anti-decubitus mattresses can also help with reducing pressure.

A mattress with several zones is best for the spine: The shoulder and pelvis areas are more elastic and give a little, while the thoracic spine can be well supported. There are mattresses with a module system so that the degree of hardness can be adjusted to the individual needs.

TIPS

✓ Individual shops offer advice and the opportunity to try out mattresses for a few days so that the best option can be found.

✓ Sheepskin can be placed in especially vulnerable places (heels, buttocks…) and a postural pillow between the knees can increase comfort and minimise pressure.

Bedclothes
The bedclothes should be able to be washed at a high temperature and dried in a dryer so that they are softer. Suitable fabrics are:
- Cotton
- DermaSilk® Microair®
- Viscose
- Flannel

Household
Children become adolescents – with a view to becoming self-sufficient later, being independent in the home should play a big role. Household activities may place a great strain on severely affected hands. The right equipment can promote independence a good deal.

Kitchen equipment
- Wheelchair access (see p. 91)
- Access below working surfaces and sink for use with a wheelchair (see Fig. 6.15)
- Easily opened drawers and doors. Tip On or Servo Drive System (with motor) – a light touch is enough to open or close
- Flat plugs, where possible, on electrical appliances are easier to take out of the socket.

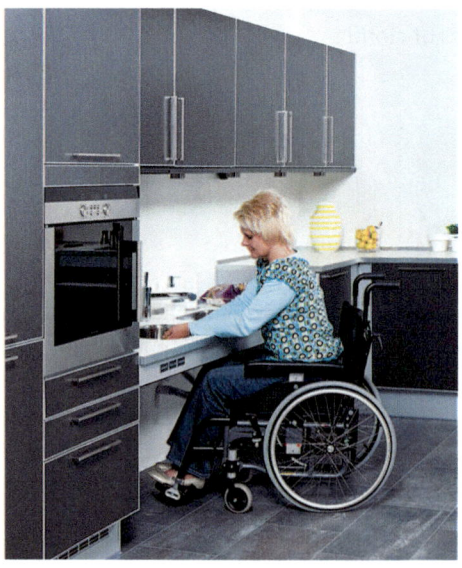

◻ **Fig. 6.15** Accessible kitchen with height-adjustable working surfaces (Ropox and Matzka Rehatechnik)

Household assistive devices
- Electric tin opener
- Special bottle and jar opener (see Fig. 6.16)
- Extra sharp serrated knife
- Chopping knife with vertical handles (mezzaluna)
- One-handed knife (Nelson) (see Fig. 6.17)

- Food processor
- Fixed brushes in the sink (see Fig. 6.18)
- Non-slip underlay
- Self-opening or table-top scissors to open packaging (see Fig. 6.30a–c)

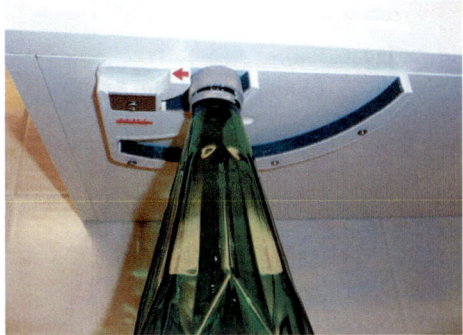

■ Fig. 6.16 Special bottle and jar opener

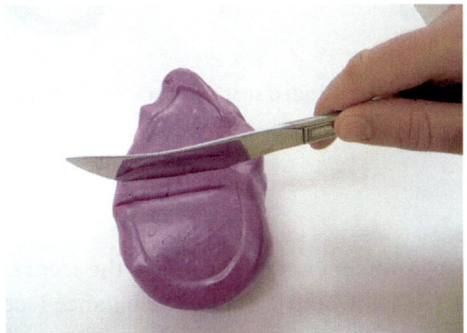

■ Fig. 6.17 One-handed knife

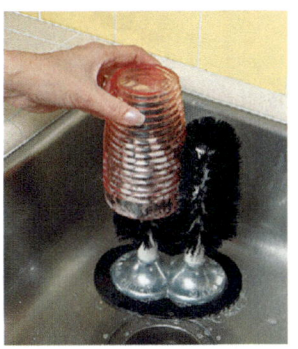

■ Fig. 6.18 Brushes in the sink
(North Coast Medical)

Front Door

The key to the front door can be on a bar (instead of a ring); by using the leverage of the bar, the door may be easily opened or locked (see Fig. 6.19).

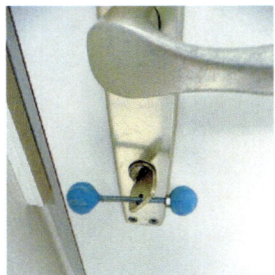

■ Fig. 6.19 Key bar

6.2.2 Mobility/Locomotion

It can be very difficult for many children to walk any distance so that using a vehicle makes it easier.

Tricycle
Ideally, the seat and backrest should be padded (see Fig. 6.20a).

Tricycle *Carry* is designed to take the affected child as passenger (see Fig. 6.20b).

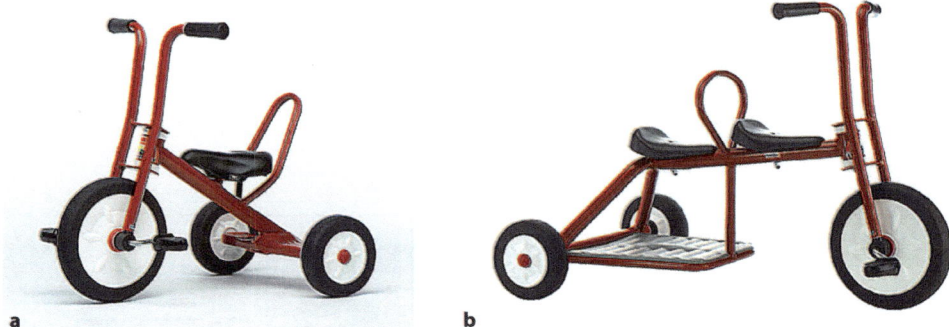

a   b

▪ **Fig. 6.20** Tricycles for children with EB. **a** Tricycle *Speedy* with padded seat and backrest (Italtrike). **b** Tricycle *Carry* (Italtrike)

Balance Bike
This enables a child to go relatively long distances independently. Because the feet remain on the ground, the danger of falling is fairly low and it trains the balance (see Fig. 6.21).

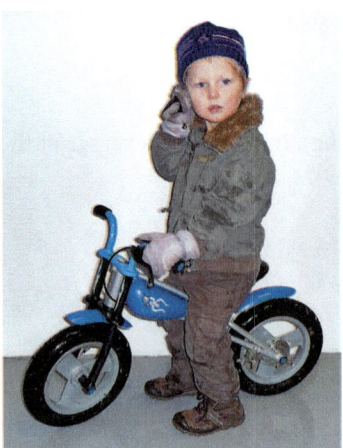

▪ **Fig. 6.21** Balance bike

Scooter
The safety scooter (see Fig. 6.22) reduces the danger of falling because of its construction. Additional safety is given by the wide wheels, wide platform and padded handles.

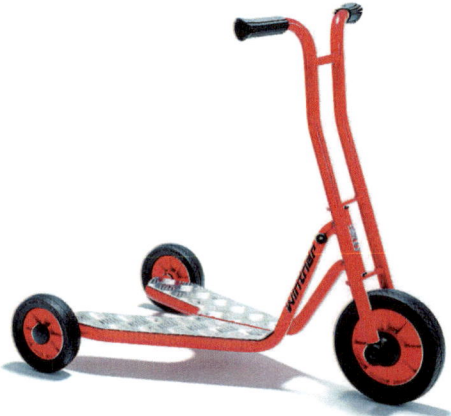

🔲 Fig. 6.22 Safety scooter (Jakobs)

Recumbent Bicycle
This bicycle is suitable for children who cannot walk. There is no need to keep balance because the vehicle stands on the ground stably (see Fig. 6.23).

The recumbent position means that no weight is taken on the arms. If the hands cannot hold the handles, loops may be added to hold the hands in place. The same can be done to the pedals for the feet.

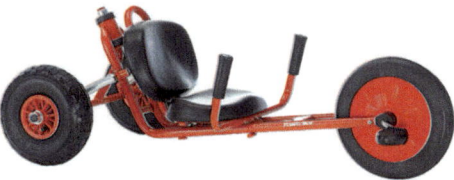

🔲 Fig. 6.23 Recumbent bicycle *Black Raider* (Italtrike)

Bicycling
The usual bicycles often provide several large challenges to persons with EB. The following changes can make it easier:
- Gel saddle
- Sheepskin cover on the saddle
- Wide moped saddle
- Back-pedalling brake if the hand brakes cannot be used
- Support wheels if necessary

- Adapted handlebars if necessary
- Smooth running gear change
- Hydraulic suspension

When a normal bicycle is insufficient, an electric bicycle or tricycle or a three-wheel electric scooter can be useful for longer distances.

Wheelchair
- Special cushion
- Electric wheelchair (see Fig. 6.24a,b)

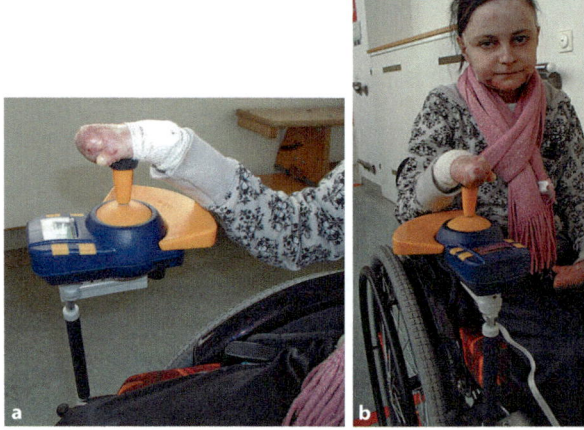

🔵 **Fig. 6.24a,b** Wheelchair adaptation for children with EB

Public Transport
Many people with EB can use public transport to some extent. An alternative is a transport service.

Car
Air conditioning is an advantage. Child seats and safety belts should be padded.

Driving a Car
There are companies that specialise in adapting cars for people with special needs. Apart from automatic gear change, there are various possibilities of changing the steering wheel so that even with poor grip it can be used (see Fig. 6.25).

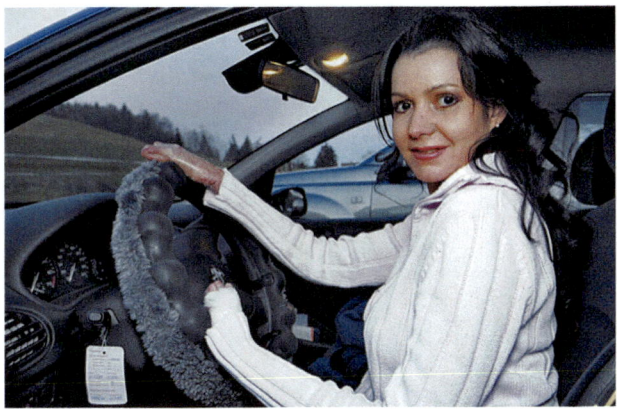

Fig. 6.25 Padded steering wheel (RDB/SI/Hervé le Cunff)

6.2.3 Leisure/Hobbies

Having a balanced leisure time is important for a good quality of life. Leisure activities assist with social integration and help raise the feeling of wellbeing because they are often done with other people.

Experience of people with EB shows they can participate in a number of hobbies and leisure activities in spite of their restrictions.

Hobbies
- Animals
- Music
- Singing
- Friends
- Drawing and painting
- Reading
- Television
- Computer games
- Handicrafts
- Dancing
- Theatre
- Photography

Participation in club life
- Choir
- Church servers
- Playgroups
- (Church) youth groups
- Football fan clubs
- Scouts

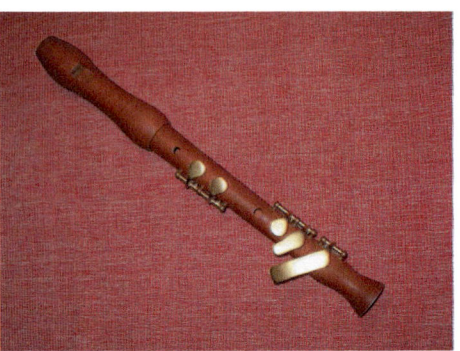

◘ **Fig. 6.26** Adapted recorder for child with finger deformities (DEBRA Austria)

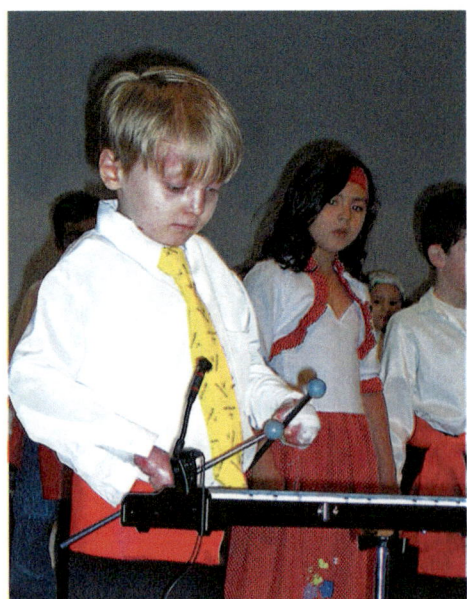

◘ **Fig. 6.27** Playing the xylophone

Sport

In the past, the idea of people with EB participating in sport was viewed differently from the current view. Great care and protection were advised. Today a few blisters will be accepted in exchange for the better physical function and quality of life.

As one affected person put it: 'All parties must end in broken bones!' (Ianina Ilitcheva).

The most popular sports are riding, swimming and cycling. However, a number of the following are also enjoyed:

- Ball games
- Gymnastics
- Inline skating
- Ice skating
- Climbing
- Skateboarding

To prevent blistering, the following measures can be taken:

- Gloves are very commonly used as protection
- Mats are spread out under equipment
- Knee protectors
- Elbow protectors

Relaxation

Recreation, relaxation and regeneration activities are important to make a change from the exertions of everyday life and pain. At home it is possible to have somewhere to retire to for peace and quiet: meditation cushions, beanbag and hammock chairs or hammocks can provide this (see Fig. 6.28a–c).

Music and massage are used by many to assist relaxation.

Television, reading and sleeping all help to distract from pain.

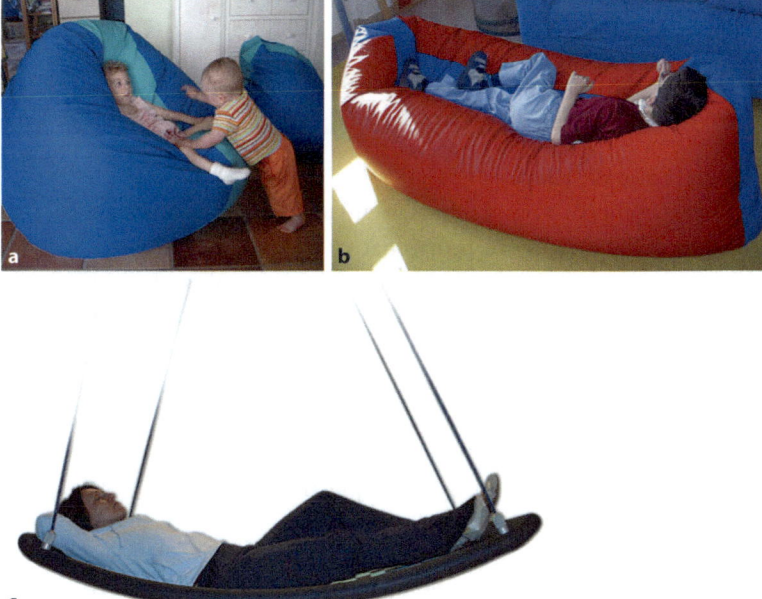

🔲 **Fig. 6.28** Relaxation suggestions. **a,b** Beanbag chairs (Matzka Rehatechnik). **c** Therapy swing (Eybl Sportbau)

Holidays

There are a number of different kinds of holidays which can be suitable depending on the conditions. The following kinds have been well proven:

- Pony club (riding)
- City trips
- Holiday homes
- Farm holidays
- Winter holidays

Beach holidays are also possible, but too much heat should be avoided because of the danger of increased blistering. A private beach can be an advantage, as it gives more protection of privacy.

Recommended conditions for holidays

- Air conditioning
- Washing machine
- Bath tub
- Possibility to purée food
- Barrier-free access (wheelchair)
- Lift
- Access with the car to transport all the necessary equipment
- Facilities for bandaging
- Assistance with luggage

6.2.4 Kindergarten (Nursery)/School/Work

Some General Comments about School

Before a child with EB starts school or nursery, it is useful to have a personal meeting with staff. The particular needs of the child in the individual situation of the school or nursery, including what special conditions are needed, can be discussed. It is also advisable to refer the teachers to some Web sites on the Internet so that they can inform themselves about the condition.

An important foundation for the integration of the child into the class is respect of the child as a person and informing the rest of the class in a sensitive manner about the situation. This can be done by giving the class information about the condition and the particular needs of the child with EB, and a question and answer session with the said child. Together consideration can be given as to how the child can contribute with his/her abilities to the class and where special attention needs to be given. Burning questions from the class about someone 'being different' can be given space and time here.

Fundamental Ideas about Inclusive Education

An effort needs to be made for the class to realise that there are differences among all children. They all learn at their own speed according to their own level of development through their joint activities, and each child has his/her own needs.

Through an open association with one another children can learn that they all profit, because each one contributes to the group and they all widen their experiences together. Everyone can profit and learn from diversity! Every child has his/her own individual strengths and weaknesses; they can all learn by being part of the community where they can develop their strengths and overcome their weaknesses. To be able to accept others with the respect one would like to have oneself is a valuable experience for life.

Group/Class Size

Generally, small groups have the advantage of there being less danger of injury and enabling more individual care.

Accompanying Persons

For children who need assistance with everyday activities, it may be possible to have teaching assistants in the classroom.

Endurance

Many people with EB have a relatively low level of endurance, because the body needs energy to cope with healing and immunity. As a result, they tire very easily and need regular breaks.

Handling

Children with EB should never be lifted up by the armpits; better is a support under the buttocks because this gives a wider area to take the weight. The second hand can then support the back of the child.

Eating at School

Either the child should take appropriate food from home or if necessary school food should be puréed. If a child needs a long time to eat, permission should be given to eat small snacks during class so that the protein and calorie intake is adequate.

School Bag or Satchel

Carrying heavy objects for a long time is very difficult for many children with EB. Alternatives are:

- Soft padding on the shoulders
- Wide straps
- Trolley instead of bag
- School bag with wheels and a handle for one hand
- A second set of books at home

TIPS

✓ Lever-arch files are easier to open.
✓ Paper binding or covers are better than plastic ones, as they do not stick to each other and so are easier to take out of the satchel.

Furnishing and Fittings

Outside

A sand pit should have not sharp corners and the sand needs to be very fine (sea sand rather than builders' sand is kinder to the skin); adequate shade with awnings is also important.

A protective surface under swings and slides helps to lower the risk of injury. Grassed areas should be without sharp stones, and bushes and trees should be cut back so that children are not hurt by branches hanging down.

Classroom
Similarly, the classroom should be suitable for a wheelchair if necessary; this includes ramps, lift, toilet and easily opened doors or electric door openers.

Gym
Usually children with EB are not expected to take part in school gym or sport, but it is important to keep in mind that there can be some activities in which it is possible for them to participate. Such physical experiences are vital for children with EB as well as the social aspect of group games. If it is not possible for them to take part, it is good if a substitute can be found, e. g. art or handicraft classes.

A Place for Bandaging
There needs to be a place for bandage and dressing materials. Bandaging needs to be done somewhere private so that others cannot see. A suitable possibility to sit and a washbasin are advantageous.

Seating in the Classroom
Best is a place in the front row to be able to follow the teaching easily and where reaching the place has the least danger of bumping into things. As heat increases blistering and the body's own heat regulation system can be affected, being close to radiators or windows where the sun shines in may be unsuitable.

To reduce the pressure of sitting for a long time, the following can be done:
- Soft chair with padding or sheepskin
- Chair seat and desk edges should be rounded

Ergonomically correct seating (see Fig. 6.29a,b) is advantageous for children with EB to develop a good upright posture and to work against the development of contractures.

The child's desk should be height-adjustable and allow the surface to be slightly sloped.
Somewhere to put books, a groove for pencils and a non-slip surface are further advantages. There should also be adequate legroom so that there are no bars to bump against, and the desk should be easily made suitable for work on a laptop.
The desk chair should be hydraulically adjustable. The feet should always rest on the floor or a footrest.
A chair with rocking bars allows some movement, which also improves concentration.
On the whole, the chair should not be too heavy so that the child with EB can move it more easily.

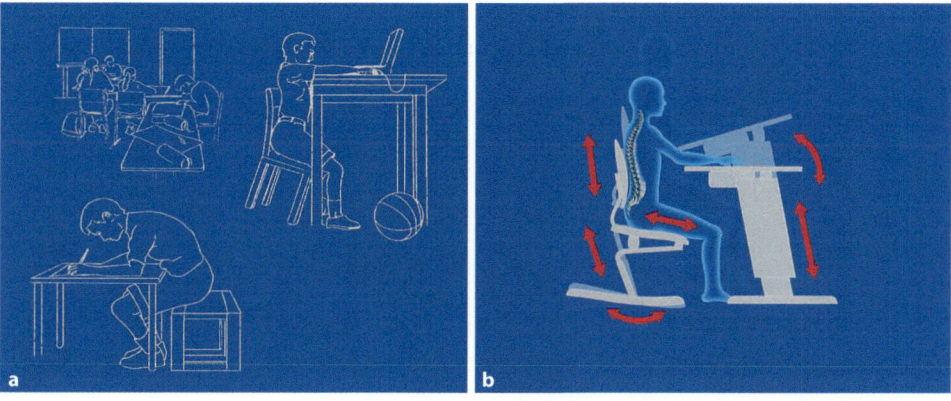

Fig. 6.29 Seating ergonomics. **a** Bad examples for sitting at a desk (AGR): 'The work place for a child: a load of stress with a 'time fuse'.' **b** Ergonomic seating (AGR): 'Commendable: The unit of desk and chair – a unity of dynamics and ergonomics!'

Handicrafts and Scissors

Using Scissors

Children with only minimal adhesions of the fingers can use ordinary children's scissors. Self-opening or easy-grip scissors (see Fig. 6.30a) give less pressure on thumb and index fingers. If the fingers have cocoon-like deformities and the thumb cannot be abducted far enough, then table-top scissors may be used (see Fig. 6.30b,c).

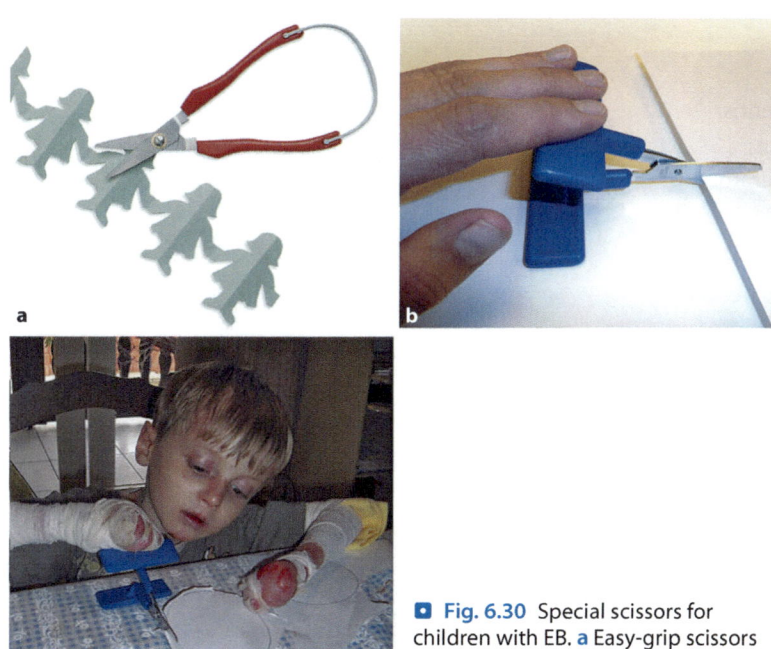

Fig. 6.30 Special scissors for children with EB. **a** Easy-grip scissors (North Coast Medical). **b** Table-top scissors. **c** Table-top scissors in use

Handicrafts

There are a number of handicrafts which most children with EB can manage to some extent, including:

- Embroidery on soft material
- Pottery
- Painting and drawing
- Knitting
- Weaving

Professional Training

Many children with EB attend ordinary schools and complete school leaving exams at either a middle level or a higher level (university entrance).

With regard to university courses there are any number of directions which may be chosen, for example:

- Art and/or history of art
- Computer studies
- Languages
- History
- Journalism and communication studies

Professional Options

Affected adolescents have mentioned, amongst others, the following career aspirations:

- Author or journalist
- Artist
- Administrator
- Computer scientist
- Mathematician
- Telephone operator
- ...

6.2.5   Barrier-Free Living

Some people with DEB need to use a wheelchair at least some of the time, so it makes sense to consider wheelchair accessibility in the home.

Accessible building is important for people with handicaps. This is needed by all wheelchair users and many elderly people. It is equally important for families with small children – prams and pushchairs need space and ramps instead of steps. It makes sense to be prepared for changes in the course of life.

Accessible building (universal design) allows for the greatest possible independence, not the least being able to visit friends and relatives as well as to access public institutions. Then there is less danger of isolation at home – 'house or room arrest'.

In many houses the passages and doorways are too narrow; toilets and bathrooms too small, and there are too many steps both in the house and at the entrance.

In newly built houses it is possible to consider aspects which make an adaptation for wheelchairs easier and not too expensive; this includes:

- Only have doors where they are absolutely necessary.
- As few weight-bearing walls as possible makes alterations later easier.
- Cooking, eating and living areas as closely as possible.
- Doors, switches, electric sockets should be at least 50 cm away from the corners.
- Electric sockets and radiator valves should be at a height easily reached from a wheelchair close.
- More electric sockets and fewer electric cables are good.
- Walls should be designed so that later grab bars or a stair lift can be added.
- Empty conduit should be laid so that electric devices can be added later (awning …).
- French windows to ensure that handles are not too high and there can be a good view from sitting positions is a good idea.

Sustainable construction allows for later cheap and quick adaptations without major changes for pipes and cables.

The standards for barrier-free building vary from country to country. Details may usually be obtained from the relevant building/planning authority.

Some examples of barrier-free design:

Car Park

The space for wheelchair users should be wider than the usual parking space. Steps should be avoided by the use of ramps, or inside there should be a lift (see Fig. 6.31a,b).

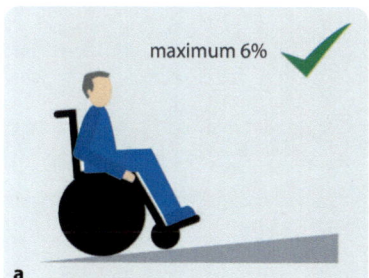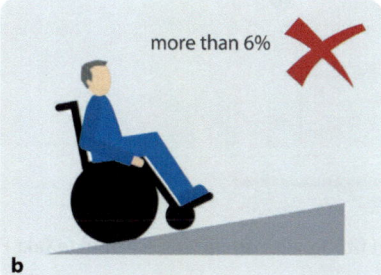

Fig. 6.31a,b The slope of a ramp for wheelchairs should not be more than 6% (eXakt PR)

6

Space for Turning

The normal space needed for a wheelchair to turn corners without bumping the wall or into other things is 1.5 m (see Fig. 6.32a–c).

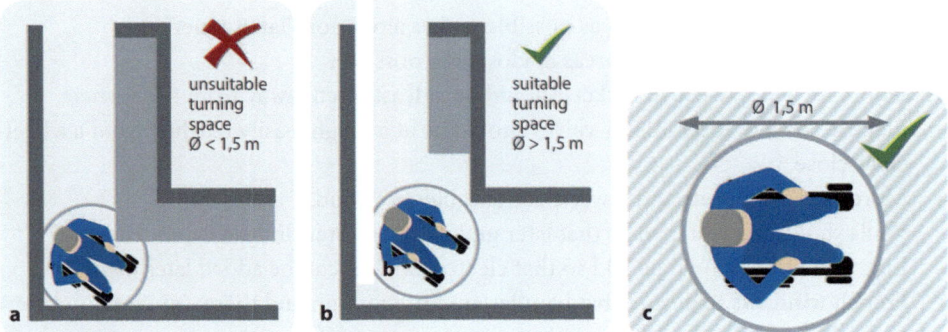

◻ **Fig. 6.32a–c** Minimum turning space for wheelchairs must have a minimum diameter of 1.5 m (eXakt PR)

Doorways

Ideally a doorway should be 90 cm wide, but it must be at least 80 cm.

Kitchen

Working surfaces should have legroom below them, and height-adjustable cabinets are advantageous (see Fig. 6.33).

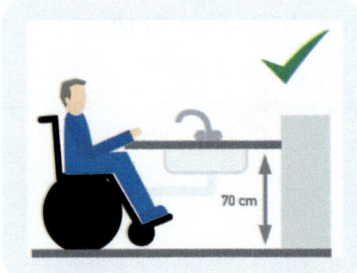

◻ **Fig. 6.33** Kitchen fitting with adequate legroom (eXakt PR)

Toilet

If a house has been designed for barrier-free living but no wheelchair is actually needed, the toilet should be rather large. This extra space can be used for storage or a washing machine. A urinal or a roll-in shower can be installed. A bidet with dryer can be installed in ordinary toilets, which can be advantageous for many people with EB, as using toilet paper is then unnecessary. Doors to toilets should either open outwards or be sliding doors.

Bedroom

The bedroom needs to be at least 3 m long. If it is 3.50 m, there is greater flexibility for placing the bed.

Window

It should be possible to see out of the window at a height of 60 cm; handles should not be higher than maximum of 1.3 m.

French windows are ideal because they have the same height as a door. From the outside there is either a small balcony or safety bars.

Barrier-free building is not usually even noticed by people; functionality can even be aesthetic (cf. Eiersebner, Prucher 2008).

7 Client-Directed Therapy Using the COSA

Florian Prinz

When working with children and youths with EB, the question arose as to how the needs and wishes of the clients could be given even more prominence in occupational therapy (OT) intervention than previously.

In the search for a client-directed therapeutic conceptual model and assessment instrument, the COSA (Child Occupational Self Assessment) seemed to meet these needs.

The assessment of children with EB aged between 8 and 13 years was then planned by using this assessment instrument, taking the special conditions and needs of these children into consideration.

7.1 Client-Directed Practice

Working in a client-directed manner means that the questions, concerns and priorities of the client are the point of reference for the therapeutic intervention. In OT this means that we must see the client as the expert for his or her own daily life (cf. Keller et al. 2006).

Thus we recognise that each person being treated knows him- or herself best and so should determine the key aspects of the intervention (cf. Jerosch-Herold et al. 2009).

The therapist gains insight into the strengths and areas of difficulty that the client perceives of him- or herself in all areas of everyday life. Using this information the client and therapist together decide on the focus, therapeutic aims and methods (cf. Pätzold et al. 2008; Keller et al. 2006).

7.2 What is COSA?

'The Child Occupational Self Assessment (COSA) is a client-directed assessment tool and an outcome measure designed to capture children's and youth's perceptions regarding their own sense of occupational competence and the importance of everyday activities' (Keller et al. 2006, p. 2). It is designed for use by children aged between 8 and 13 years. By using the COSA the child can gain an insight into his/her own strengths and problems. The therapist is able to plan the intervention with the client on equal terms.

The COSA was developed by Keller et al. and later translated into German by Pätzold et al. (2008); in doing so some additions were made which have proved to be very useful for children with EB. Prinz has made some more additions specifically for children with EB. All these additions are referred to below.

7.2.1 Contents and Structure of the COSA

The COSA (version 2.1) consists of 25 items which the child marks independently by using the given symbols of smileys and stars. To make it easier for the reader to understand, the items 1–5 of the self-assessment form are shown in Fig. 7.1. The child's answers give information as to how he/she perceives his/her activity performance (smileys), e. g. 'I have a big problem doing this' or 'I am really good at doing this'. Marking the stars allows the child to express interests, priorities and values.

Estimating the value of an activity highlights those areas where the child is satisfied or dissatisfied with his/her performance.

Myself	I have a big problem doing this	I have a little problem doing this	I do this ok	I am really good at doing this	Not really important to me	Important to me	Really important to me	Most important of all to me
Keep my body clean	☹ ☹	☹	☺	☺ ☺	☆	☆ ☆	☆ ☆ ☆	☆ ☆ ☆ ☆
Dress myself	☹ ☹	☹	☺	☺ ☺	☆	☆ ☆	☆ ☆ ☆	☆ ☆ ☆ ☆
Eat my meals without any help	☹ ☹	☹	☺	☺ ☺	☆	☆ ☆	☆ ☆ ☆	☆ ☆ ☆ ☆
Buy something myself	☹ ☹	☹	☺	☺ ☺	☆	☆ ☆	☆ ☆ ☆	☆ ☆ ☆ ☆
Get my chores done	☹ ☹	☹	☺	☺ ☺	☆	☆ ☆	☆ ☆ ☆	☆ ☆ ☆ ☆

🔹 **Fig. 7.1** Items 1–5 of the self-assessment form (Keller et al. 2006, p. 29)

The *'Intended Meaning Reference Guide'* can be used to further clarify the meaning of the COSA statements when a child needs it. It also gives a good overview of the 25 items of the self-assessment form, at the end of which there are also three open questions. These give the child additional possibilities of expressing him-/herself regarding any other strengths or problems he/she may have in his/her occupational competence.

After the COSA has been completed, the child and therapist interpret and discuss the results together and identify the strengths and problems of the child. At the end of the discussion they decide together which areas the child would most like to change. In this way the therapist and client together establish treatment goals. A time is also recorded by when a goal is to be achieved. A follow-up should be completed 3–6 months after intervention, and this will establish whether the goals have been attained (cf. Keller et al. 2006).

As children live in close context with their families/parents, an extended version of the COSA was made in German as mentioned above. In this version the parents may fill out the form at the same time but independently of the child and in another room. It is then possible to discuss the opinions of both parents and child, and this may flow into the planning of the intervention (cf. Pätzold et al. 2008).

COSA Intended Meaning Reference Guide

COSA Statements	Intended Meaning
Keep my body clean	You are able to wipe or wash your hands and face. You take a shower or bath without any help. You brush your teeth and hair by yourself.
Dress myself	You are able choose what you want to wear and are able to put your clothes on without any help.
Eat my meals without any help	You are able use a fork, spoon, and knife to eat with, and a cup or glass to drink from without spilling or needing any help.
Buy something myself	You are able choose an item to buy and know how much money to give to a cashier. If you had a dollar, you would know how to purchase a needed or desired item. The purchase could take place within school, the community, or any other setting.
Get my chores done	You are able to finish jobs asked of you without any help from others. Chores could involve hobs assigned in the home, classroom, or other setting as appropriate.
Get enough sleep	You sleep enough so that you have the energy to do the things you need or want to do.
Have enough time to do things I like	You keep a good schedule to get your work done so you have free-time to do things you like to do.
Take care of my things	You keep your clothes, books, games, and other things neatly so that you can easily find what you need.
Get around from one place to another	You cane move your entire body to get to where you need to go. (This item refers to mobility within the client's various environments rather than gross motor skills.)
Choose things that I want to do	You can choose things you want to do to have fun. You have the control to choose one activity over another in an appropriate situation. (For example, you cannot choose to not finish your class work, but you can choose what activities you can do within reason during free time.)
Keep my mind on what I'm doing	You are able to keep thinking about what you are doing. You do not need someone to remind you to finish.
Do things with my family	You are able to work and play with the members of your family.
Do things with my friends	You have others your age that you like to be with and do things with.
Do things with my classmates	You are able to get along with the children in your class to work and share in school.
Follow classroom rules	You understand and follow the rules and schedule of your classroom.
Finish my work in class on time	You are able to start your class work once your teacher asks you to and you keep working at it so you finish on time.
Get my homework done	You are able study at home to finish your homework on time.
Ask my teacher questions when I need to	You are able to ask your teacher for help when you do not understand something or when you have having a problem.
Make others understand my ideas	You are able to share your thoughts and feelings so others understand.
Think of ways to do things when I have a problem	You try other ways of doing things when you are having difficulty.
Keep working on something even when it gets hard	You keep working on what you are doing even if it is hard.
Calm myself down when I am upset	You can stop feeling angry, sad, or frustrated when something bad happens. You know things you can do to help mad, sad or frustrated feelings go away.
Make my body do what I want it to do	You can make your body move to play, work and do the things you want to do. (This item refers to gross motor skills.)
Use my hands to work with things	You can make your hands and fingers move to do things with games, school supplies, or other objects.
Finish what I am doing without getting tired too soon	You get done with what you are doing without your body needing to rest.

Fig. 7.2 COSA *Intended Meaning Reference Guide* (Keller et al. 2006, p. 10–11)

7.3 Client-Directed Assessment and Therapy for Children with EB Using the COSA

Using the COSA for children with EB, it very soon became apparent that some additions were needed, e. g. extending some explanations to the items or adding more items.

Some items of the COSA are not very relevant for the assessed children with EB. Children have the freedom to leave out non-relevant items, so that that there was no need to remove them from the assessment. They might still be relevant to other children and also most of the less relevant items were marked with 'I do this OK' or 'I am really good at doing this'. It is important for children and youths with EB to have some items that they can mark in this way, as there are a great many items, especially those concerning physical abilities (movement, mobility, dexterity) that may be expected to have a negative evaluation. The children experience that there are areas in which they are very good alongside the many items that without question present difficulties. They are able to have a new view of their resources and are then not only concerned with their deficits.

The discussion of the self-assessment results with the children has been shown to be extremely important. The child should express his/her thoughts and judgement about each of the items. The therapist notes the issues which, according to the child and his/her personal situation, abilities and environmental conditions, lead to difficulties (cf. Pätzold et al. 2008; Keller et al. 2006).

Because many issues specific to the condition of EB are the cause of problems, the discussion between the therapist and the child is a vital basis for the analysis of problems and planning of the intervention. The therapist learns more details as to why an item was marked in the way it was.

For example, item 7, 'Have enough time to do things I like', was marked by the child 'I have a little problem doing this'. The value scale was marked 'most important of all to me'. In the discussion it turned out that the daily changing of bandages took 2 h, and eating also needed a long time because of the problems with the oesophagus. There was less time left for other activities.

During the discussion it can happen that the child discovers other aspects or changes his/her mind and so alters the evaluation which is perfectly acceptable.

7.3.1 Additions to the *Intended Meaning Reference Guide* for Children with EB

It has proved useful to extend or reformulate some of the intended meanings; these are listed here.

Intended Meaning for Item 3, 'Eat my Meals without any Help'
'You are able use a fork, spoon, and knife to eat with, and a cup or glass to drink from without spilling or needing any help'.

To which has been added, 'You can make yourself a snack' in the German version, and 'Cut soft food with a knife' for children with EB.

Intended Meaning for Item 4, 'Buy Something myself'

'You are able choose an item to buy and know how much money to give to a cashier. If you had a dollar, you would know how to purchase a needed or desired item. The purchase could take place within school, the community, or any other setting'.

For children with EB, 'You can take money out of your purse and use it to pay' has been added.

Intended Meaning for Item 5, 'Get my Chores Done'

'You are able to finish jobs asked of you without any help from others. Chores could involve jobs assigned in the home, classroom, or other setting as appropriate'.

For children with EB it states, 'You are able to finish jobs asked of you without any help from others *in as far as you are physically able to*. Chores could involve jobs assigned in the home, classroom or other setting, as appropriate.'

Intended Meaning for Item 7, 'Have Enough Time to Do Things I Like'

'You keep a good schedule to get your work done so you have free-time to do things you like to do.'

For children with EB this has been extended to state, 'You keep a good schedule to get your work done *and also when all the jobs of the day like changing bandages, getting dressed, eating, homework etc. are done,* you have enough free-time to do things you like to do.'

Intended Meaning for Item 9, 'Get Around from One Place to Another'

'You can move your entire body to get to where you need to go.'

The German translation of COSA was slightly extended for this item and for children with EB this is also recommended. It states, 'You can move your entire body, *with or without wheelchair, bicycle or bus* to get to where you need to go.' (cf. Pätzold et al. 2008).

Intended Meaning for Item 16, 'Finish my Work in Class on Time'

'You are able to start your class work once your teacher asks you to and you keep working at it so you finish on time.'

For children with EB this has been extended to state, 'You are able to start your class work once your teacher asks you to, *you can work fast enough and* you keep working at it so you finish on time.'

This is because most affected children have severe restrictions to their dexterity and so often work much slower.

7.3.2   Additional Items for Children with EB

The following items have been added for children with EB because experience has shown that they are valuable to them.

'I Can Carry the Things I Need'

The intended meaning is, 'You can carry the things you need at school or at home without help (e.g. school bag/satchel, school books, lunch box, bottle …).'

'I Can Go on Holiday/Vacation'

The intended meaning is, 'You and your family can go away for a few days, or you can take part in a school outing lasting a few days.'

'I Can Care for my Blisters/Sores myself'

(for Children from the Age of 10 Years)

The intended meaning is, 'You can change bandages and dress sores on those parts of your body you can reach.'

7.3.3   Formulating Goals

It is important to take into consideration that in some forms of EB (especially DEB) there will be only very little if any progress in some areas because of the advancing nature of the condition (e.g. webbing – even after surgical finger separation new webbing may form within 3 to 5 years).

When formulating goals therapist and client together can therefore give priority to maintaining specific abilities for as long as possible (e.g. by using splinting, bandaging and exercises after operations over a long period to prevent or retard webbing for as long as possible).

There are areas where it must sometimes be accepted that no change of the physical or EB-specific conditions is possible.

Example: Item 25, 'Finish what I am doing without getting tired too soon.'

Children with EB often get tired much sooner than non-affected children, because the healing process requires a great deal of energy, and so there is a tendency for their entire body to be weakened.

In this case, the planning of the intervention can include whether it is possible to make changes to the situation or to the environment to ease the problem. For example, some of the following measures can help:

- Split tiring tasks into smaller steps (pacing).
- Make short breaks before becoming tired.
- Carry out relaxation exercises in the breaks for an effective revival.
- Economise on the steps in the job so that the task causes less strain.
- Structure the work environment so that those other aspects unrelated to the condition, like noise, lighting, indoor climate or constricted space, which cause strain are reduced etc.

Example: Item 7, 'Have enough time to do things I like.'

As mentioned above, changing bandages and eating often take up a great deal of time in some forms of EB, which is then not available for other activities. These tasks must be done but it can be considered whether they could be organised somewhat better:

- Eat small portions several times a day to consume the necessary calories and to avoid extended meal times.
- Eat while watching television or playing computer games – the activity distracts from pain on swallowing and the time is being used for leisure activities.

Looking at the goals that the children and youths with EB choose, it becomes apparent that items are also chosen which are less dependent on the condition EB, e.g. item 22, 'Calm myself down when I am upset'. This shows that these children are not only concerned with their physical state, but are also occupied with such psychosocial aspects that affect other children as well.

8 Rehabilitation of the Hand

Hedwig Weiß

8.1 Pathophysiology of the Hand

Each type of epidermolysis bullosa (EB) is characterised by a fragility of the epithelial layers, blistering due to mechanical force and poorly healing sores.

Mitten-like contractures and deformities of the hands and the feet are present in nearly all patients with the sub-type Hallopeau-Siemens, a recessive dystrophic type of epidermolysis bullosa (RDEB). Most of the EB patients in occupational therapy (OT) who require hand rehabilitation have this type (see Fig. 8.1). In other types, such as dominant dystrophic, junctional and simplex, the number of patients who develop deformities is much lower (cf. Fine et al. 2005).

It has become apparent that, apart from the dystrophic symptoms of the skin, the bones have a lower density than normal. Fewtrell et al. (2006) have found that children with recessive dystrophic and junctional EB are affected by this reduction in bone density, and so are more likely to suffer splintered fractures. The causes would appear to be multiple; specific research is necessary to find out more. The authors propose the hypothesis that increased activity and so using the bones can have a preventative effect for these children. It is unfortunately a fact that increased physical exercise for those with RDEB sub-type Hallopeau-Siemens is extremely difficult because of the severity of the condition. With other types, some degree of strengthening is easier because the deformities are less serious and the whole metabolism of the skin is better.

This knowledge underlines the importance of physical exercise as more than just contracture prophylaxis for the joints; it also improves the general metabolism and the strength of the bones. Muscle activity also stimulates and improves the development of bone density.

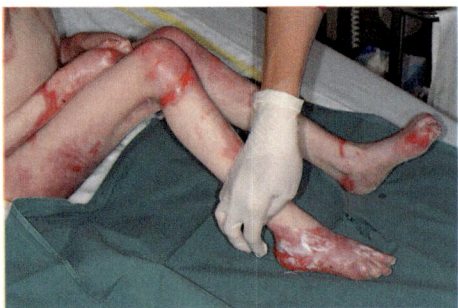

◘ **Fig. 8.1** The state of the skin of a patient with DEB. Hand and foot deformities (Hametner)

8.2 Contractures and Deformities

In this section the deformities of the hands which are most common in RDEB type Hallopeau-Siemens are described because they present the biggest need for therapeutic intervention. Patients with such severe deformities of the hands are extremely handicapped in their activities of daily life and so are the main people referred to OT. Prophylactic splinting, bandaging or use of compression gloves and exercise should help to delay the development of contractures and deformities.

Pseudosyndactyly starts to develop very gradually from infancy and by the age of 20 years; 98 % of those who have the sub-type Hallopeau-Siemens have this problem (cf. Fine et al. 2005). The cause is a lengthening of the commissure (web space) from proximal to distal, a process called webbing.

Pseudosyndactyly is typified by a fusion of all fingers; isolated movement of the fingers is no longer possible. Sometimes a certain amount of movement of the thumb is retained because it gets used so much, whereas spreading the fingers out (abduction) is completely lost (see Fig. 8.2a).

In comparison, only 3 % of patients with the dominant dystrophic type show these changes by the age of 40 years. Seventeen per cent of patients with JEB-Herlitz are affected by the age of 15 years, and 9 % with JEB-non-Herlitz by the age of 45 years (cf. Fine et al. 2005).

Flexion contractures of the fingers develop along with the webbing (see Fig. 8.2b); this reduces the finger flexion and extension or even makes it impossible.

In congenital syndactyly the adhesions of differently long fingers often limit the growth and may even cause a rotation fault of the bones of the longer finger. Clinical observations indicate that these symptoms are most likely also present in the pseudosyndactyly of people with EB. Postoperatively the scarring or poor healing of the wounds can cause contractures and possibly skeletal changes. Several patterns of contractures develop, but it is difficult to classify them as the different types overlap with each other.

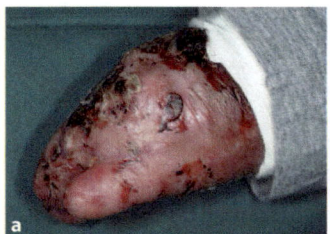 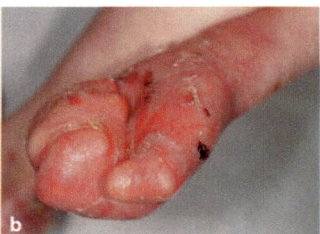

■ Fig. 8.2 a Pseudosyndactyly (Hametner). b Finger contractures with webbing (mitten-like glove) (Hametner)

8.2.1 Fingers

Some examples of the contracture patterns are now described.

One form affects mainly the proximal interphalangeal joints (PIP); the distal interphalangeal joints (DIP) remain free. At the same time, a contracture of the adductors (adductor pollicis, interosseus dorsalis I) of the first metacarpal (MC I) is present (see Fig. 8.3a,b).

In another variation, the flexion contracture of the fingers starts distally. The first flexion contracture begins in the DIP joints and if it spreads to the PIP joints, then a claw hand deformity develops with the fingers becoming fixed into a hook position. The extrinsic extensors which keep the MCP joints in extension become shortened.

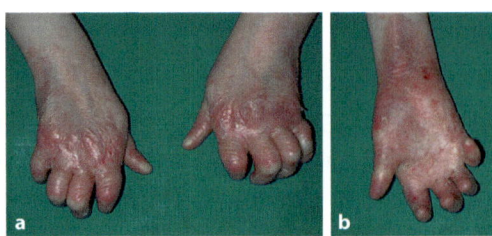

◘ **Fig. 8.3 a** Contractures of the PIP joints. **b** Contractures of the adductors and the MC I

When contractures of the fingers and pseudosyndactylies develop, there is an increased shortening of the extrinsic extensors causing hyperextension of the MCP joints and a weakening of the intrinsic muscles. The fingers are thus fixed in a hook grip position. The webbing also prevents the interossei from being active (see Fig. 8.4a,b).

In the thumb the adductor pollicis brevis becomes shorter and so its antagonist, the abductor pollicis brevis, becomes weaker. In addition the opponens pollicis muscle may become relatively inadequate.

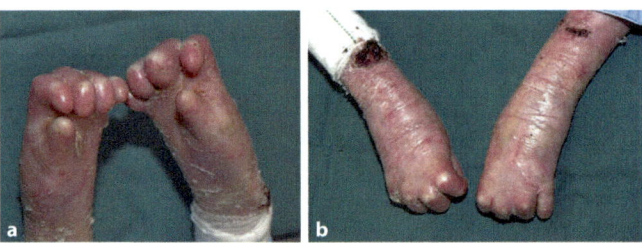

◘ **Fig. 8.4 a** Contracture into a hook grip (palmar). **b** Contracture into a hook grip (dorsal). Webbing up to the PIP joints

The flexion contractures can develop further towards a full fist, but here the degree may be different for each finger (see Fig. 8.5a,b). It can also be observed that contractures tend to start on the ulnar side and the radial fingers are mostly affected later (cf. Mullett 1998). One cause for this development could be that daily life forces more fine motor functions, which can be achieved with a three-point precision grip. The greater use of the first three digits – the more dynamic digits – may delay the development of the deformity. The ring and little finger are more static because they are used more for holding things. A biomechanical explanation may be the loss of tension of the transverse arch starting from the ulnar side (see Fig. 8.6).

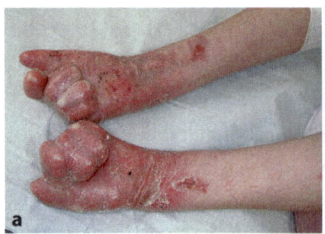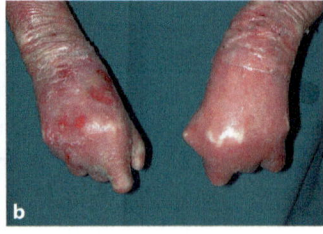

◘ **Fig. 8.5 a** Contracture into a fist (palmar). **b** Contracture into a fist (dorsal). Differing degrees of contracture of the fingers

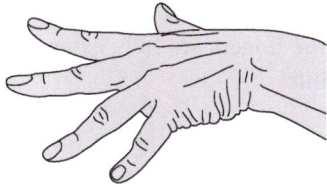

◻ **Fig. 8.6** Transverse arches of the hand (© Hochschild 2005, p. 195)

Another contracture pattern is a flexion contracture of the MCP joints with almost fully extended interphalangeal joints (IP). This looks like a lumbrical position with shortened lumbricals, which provoke the pattern (see Fig. 8.7a,b).

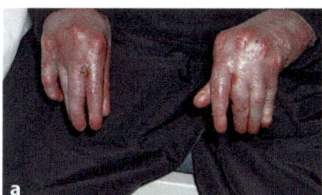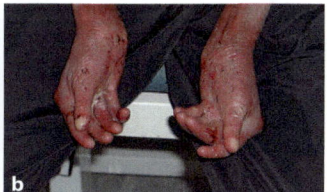

◻ **Fig. 8.7 a** Contracture in the lumbrical position. **b** Minimal contractures of the IP joint

8.2.2 Thumb

An adduction contracture, and in further advanced cases, pseudo-opposition contracture develops in the thumb so that the entire MC I is pulled in adduction and pseudo-opposition towards the MC II (see Fig. 8.8a,b).

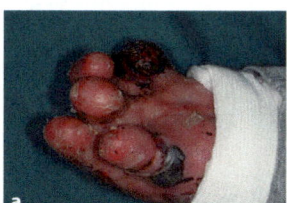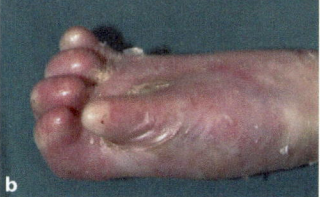

◻ **Fig. 8.8 a** Adduction contracture of the thumb. **b** Adduction contracture – pseudo-opposition contracture

A hyperextension of the MCP often develops in compensation. To be able to hold objects, the thumb has to be abducted and extended; due to the enormous restriction of radial and palmar abduction of the thumb there has to be more movement in the MCP joint – hyperextension is the result. Almost the entire opening to grasp has to come from the MCP joint. A secondary problem of this hyperextension may be instability and a subluxation of the MCP. A contracture of the adductor pollicis brevis, the opponens pollicis and the first dorsal interosseus develops (cf. Mullett 1998).

Added to this, there are contractures of the neurovascular sheaths of the fingers (cf. Ludwikowski 2009); this results in ischaemia as soon as the fingers are fully extended. This must be considered when providing night resting splints!

8.2.3 Palm and Arches of the Hand

The position of the palm of the hand and the hand arches is related to the finger contractures. When the fingers are fixed in flexion at the PIP and DIP joints forming a claw hand and the MCP joints are fixed in extension, then there is an automatic flattening of the transverse arches. If the finger contractures include the MCP joints and are stronger on the ulnar side of the hand than on the radial side, then the transverse arch is pulled towards ulnar because the ligaments of MCP IV and V provide most of the movement (see Fig. 8.9).

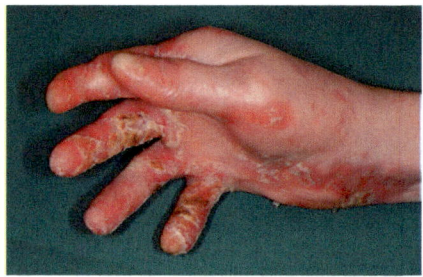

■ **Fig. 8.9** Flexion contracture starting at ulnar and pulling the transverse arch towards MCP IV and V

8.2.4 Wrist

Flexion contractures begin in the fingers and often spread to the wrist causing some degree of flexion contracture with ulnar deviation (see Fig. 8.10a,b).

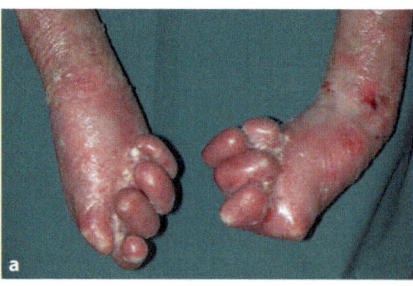

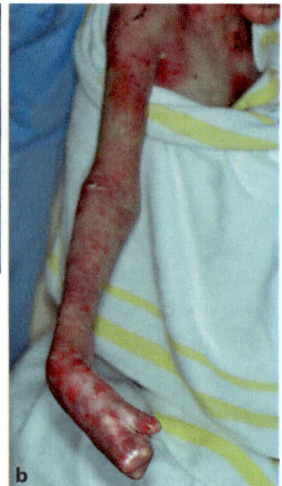

■ **Fig. 8.10 a** Flexion contracture of the wrist with ulnar deviation. **b** Extreme flexion contracture of the wrist (Hametner)

Biomechanically, the pattern of the contracture can be explained by the shape of the radio-ulnar joint surface, which slopes diagonally towards ulnar, so providing the tendency towards an ulnar deviation. The dorsopalmar angle of the joint surface of 10–20° encourages flexed position (see Fig. 8.11). The main cause of the flexion contracture is probably the posture adopted due to blistering and to relieve the resulting pain. In this position the strength of the flexors is dominant.

As a secondary complication, this relieving posture causes certain muscle groups such as flexor carpi ulnaris to predominate.

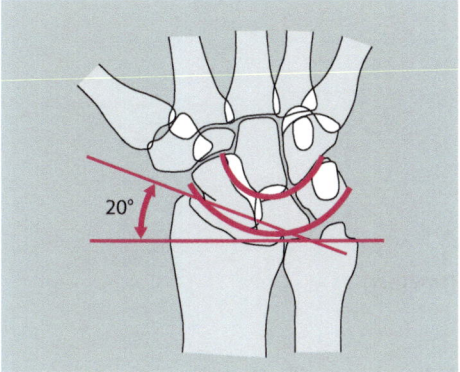

■ **Fig. 8.11** Radio-ulnar joint surface (© Hochschild 2005, p. 170)

8.2.5 Interdigital Spaces

Parallel to the limitations of motion, the development of webbing (see p. 105) gives the fingers the appearance of having become shorter. This affects the thumb a good deal as well. However, it can be observed that even in the most serious contractures, the thumb remains mobile at least from the IP joint so that objects can be held between the thumb and the fist.

The adhesions of the fingers can form the hand into a mitten, and this is surrounded by an epidermal cocoon (see Fig. 8.12). Inside this cocoon the fingers can be moved a very small amount; some patients experience this as feeling trapped inside their own body.

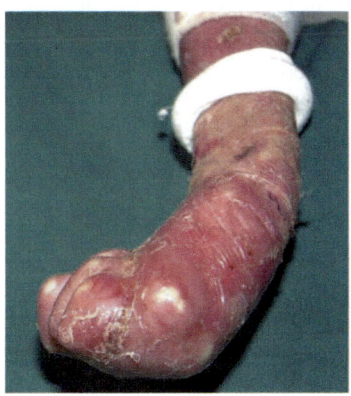

■ **Fig. 8.12** Epidermal cocoon

The resulting lack of movement in turn leads to contractures of the extrinsic and intrinsic muscles. Further the bone density, which is already poorer than in people without EB, loses more substance resulting in osteoporotic changes, which may even go as far as resorption of the bone matrix (cf. Fine et al. 2005).

It can also be observed that hands which have been cocoon-like mittens for a long time and are then operated on are still deformed. The MCP joints show a tendency towards ulnar deviation. The cause of this is not clear (see Fig. 8.13).

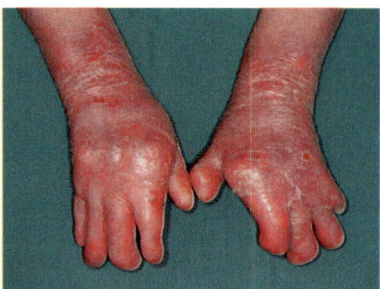

□ **Fig. 8.13** Ulnar deviation of the MCP joints left (Hametner)

8.2.6 Causes of Contractures and their Relevance to Daily Life

Both hands, dominant and non-dominant, are equally affected. It is not clear to what extent injuries and the resulting sores and scars play a role in the development of contractures. It is unlikely that they are the only cause. In any case blisters and sores in certain areas lead to protective and relieving postures, which may be further encouraged by bandaging, and all this promotes restrictions to movement.

This limited movement makes it more difficult to carry out the ordinary activities of self-care that are necessary. Children are hindered in exploring and experiencing their environment. Bandages, which are necessary in certain places because of blisters, or gloves as webbing prophylaxis, prevent the experience of tactile stimulation on the entire hand. Usually only the fingers are uncovered and able to feel. Furthermore contractures of the fingers are a strong influence on play because certain objects or toys cannot be manipulated. It can however also be observed that even with cocoon-like mittens it is possible to hold a writing implement, though the stamina for writing is extremely limited.

Separating the fingers and reducing the flexion contractures surgically is one way of increasing the ability to grasp (cf. Ludwikowski 2009).

8.2.7 Pathological Changes to the Joints Due to Contractures

Animal experiments have shown that muscles atrophy in a very short time when immobilised, and there are fibrous fatty changes in the connective tissue of joints. Within 10 days, the joint capsule loses tension, resulting in changes to the mechanics and stability of the joint.

The joint capsule then begins to shrink, and after 30 days there are adhesions between the capsule tissue and the cartilage. The cartilage then gradually shrinks and becomes thinner. After 60 days there is the beginning of pressure necrosis on the joint surfaces which are pressed together because of the fixed position. There are biochemical and structural changes in the capsule and the ligaments, tendons and fascia. The direction of the fibres changes so that cross-links are built and the elasticity and resilience of the tissue is reduced (cf. Mink et al. 2001).

8.3 Radiological Changes

Greider and Flatt (1998) mention the different changes which can be seen with X-rays: Hand and foot deformities with a generalised osteoporosis, wedge-shaped narrowing and hook-shaped changes to the distal phalanges, narrowed and constricted bones, osteolysis of the acra, flexion contractures, metatarsophalangeal (MTP) and metacarpophalangeal (MCP) subluxation, disappearance of the first interdigital space, and covering of the contracted fingers with a cocoon or mitten. Apart from this, delays in the skeletal development, bony stiffening, for example in the proximal IP joints, resorption of the heads of the metatarsals and metacarpals, shortened metatarsal bones, carpal and tarsal fusions and destruction as well as cystic changes of radius and ulna have all been observed.

These deformities of the hands, which are usually a progressive development, lead to more and more limitations, less fine motor function, dexterity and less ability to grasp and hold (see Fig. 8.14a,b).

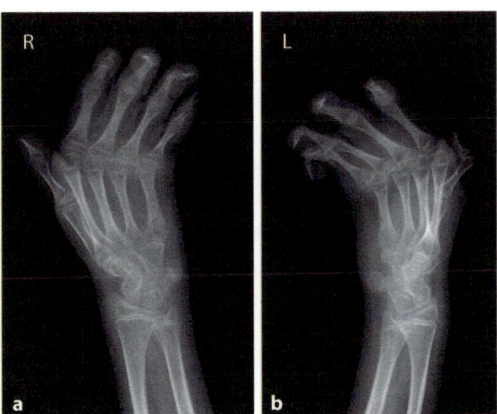

◘ Fig 8.14 a Ulnar drift of the MCP joints and bony fusion of the IP joint (SALK). b Ulnar drift and subluxation of the MCP joints (SALK)

8.4   Surgical Procedures

Ludwikowski (2009) describes that it could be possible to use various surgical procedures; the choice and execution lies in the judgement of the individual surgeon. The adduction contracture of the thumb is usually released with deep palmar and dorsal incisions in the first commissure. The finger contractures are separated by sharp, X-shaped incisions on the palmar side, between the PIP and DIP joints. The fingers are then extended and the tendons stretched. Through the stretching of the vessels the blood supply is affected, so the healing takes longer than usual and the danger of infection is increased. The use of artificial skin is controversial and is being discussed. It is often used in secondary trauma of the hands and fingers.

Postoperatively, an antiseptic cream is used to prevent infection and non-stick dressings are applied. Finally, the hand is placed in a palmar plaster longuette, with the wrist in the neutral position or in slight dorsal extension, the fingers in extension and the thumb in abduction and extension. It is important to place the wrist and fingers in the correct axis. For the first 2 weeks, the dressings are changed about every 2–5 days, depending on the severity of the operation and the healing process, using a brief general anaesthetic to prevent trauma to the child from the appalling pain and the sight of the wounds. Thereafter, dressings are changed without anaesthetic; they are often softened in a bath of Betaisodona,[1] and usually the patient removes them him- or herself in arduous, protracted, detailed work (see Fig. 8.15).

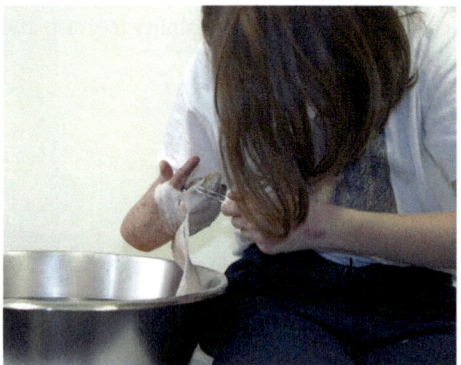

◘ Fig. 8.15 Changing the dressing (Hametner)

During the changing of dressings, time is used to carry out a few finger exercises. On the whole, a few wobbly movements of the individual fingers can be performed without the bandaging when the incisions are not fully healed. The wrist usually has more movement. During the healing process or once the operated area is healed, thermoplastic splints are made. They have the advantage that they can be easily altered and they are lightweight. After about 4 to 6 weeks the wounds on the hands have usually healed. During this time,

---

1   A disinfectant containing providone–iodine.

the splints should be worn day and night, and only taken off when doing finger exercises. Once the healing is complete a change is made to using night resting splints. Sometimes these may be worn during the day, as the skin is so extremely hypersensitive to touch that splints can be a protection against unpleasant contact.

The operation is only meaningful if it is carried out in conjunction with the splinting; otherwise new contractures develop within a few months. For this reason, good cooperation between surgeon and therapist is essential. By using the night resting splints consistently, further development of contractures may be delayed for as long as possible. The usual period between operations is 2–3 years (see Fig. 8.16a–c).

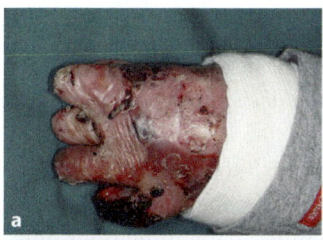
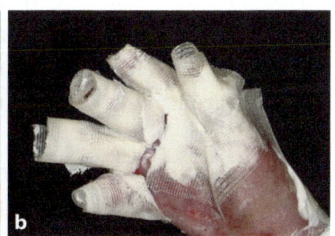
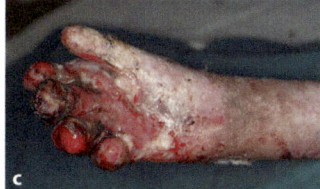

◘ **Fig. 8.16** **a** Hand of a DEB patient before the operation (Hametner). **b** Hand of the same DEB patient after the operation, with dressings (Hametner). **c** Hand of the same DEB patient after the operation (Hametner)

8.5   Occupational Therapy Process

Evidence-Based Medicine

The therapeutic intervention should follow the principles of evidence-based medicine (EBM) or evidence-based practice (EBP).

EBM is the conscientious, assertive and responsible use of the best scientific evidence available for decision-making for the care of the individual patient. For clinical practice that means formulating a problem relevant to the therapeutic situation and searching the medical literature for articles that are concerned with this problem. Those results showing relevant evidence are then applied and these results re-evaluated (cf. Koesling, Bollinger Herzka 2008).

Clinical Reasoning

Clinical reasoning is the systematic structuring of the therapeutic thought processes. In this way, the therapist should be in a position to use his or her competencies in the therapeutic situation correctly and, at the same time, to reflect on this so as to continually improve his or her therapeutic competence (cf. Koesling, Bollinger Herzka 2008).

8.6   Occupational Therapy Intervention

Experience shows that the first flexion contractures of the fingers or the first abduction deficit of the thumb begins when the child is about 4 years old. At this time, children are referred to OT, to be supplied with night resting splints to delay the process of change as far and as long as possible. An exercise programme should be given additionally to support the splinting. If surgery is indicated, the occupational therapist will have the job of postoperative splinting as soon as the plaster is removed. Again exercises should complement the splinting. An explanation of splinting, postoperative splinting and the different types of splints which can be used for contracture prophylaxis are discussed in their own section (see Chaps. 8.8.3 and 4). Often children wish to learn to play a musical instrument and to participate in subjects at school which require fine motor dexterity and good coordination. To make this possible, the parents have to make the decision to have surgery to release the adhesions.

Especially during puberty adolescents have a very strong wish to have 'normal hands' instead of fingers which have grown into a mitten. They often have the necessary motivation to undergo an operation and to cope with all the difficulties: pain, limitations of the activities of daily living and being unable to write, etc.

Compression gloves with padding in the palm are often recommended to help prevent webbing. They also offer some protection as well as supporting the transverse arches.

Modified bandaging, as done for people with rheumatoid arthritis (cf. Bitzer, Sörensen 2010), helps to influence the webbing and the ulnar deviation of the fingers at the same time.

8.7   Occupational Therapy Assessment

During the initial interview, information is noted about the development of the condition and all treatment and procedures to date. The patient should explain his or her own motivation for the OT intervention.

It is then necessary to observe any relieving postures, avoidance or evasion behaviours, malpositions and particular postures, for example during play.

An analysis of this follows, and from this the aims of the intervention can be set in discussion with the patient to meet his or her needs and to ensure a client-centred approach.

In the following section various assessment instruments are described which can be used as appropriate.

8.7.1   Assessment Form for the Hand – Using the AO Neutral-0 Method

The AO neutral-0 method is standard in hand rehabilitation. It is an exact instrument to document the range of motion.

ASSESSMENT FORM – HAND
AO neutral-0 method

Patient:	Date of birth:
Date:	Tel.:
Diagnosis:	
Date of surgery:	Therapist:
School/profession:	Doctor:
Dominance: ☐ right ☐ left	
Special notes:	
Aims of intervention:	

Measurement		Date:						Date:				
Wrist ex/flex	r.	/	/					/	/			
	l.	/	/					/	/			
Sup/pro	r.	/	/					/	/			
	l.	/	/					/	/			
Ulnar/rad. dev.	r.	/	/					/	/			
	l.	/	/					/	/			
Fingers/thumb		I	II	III	IV	V		I	II	III	IV	V
Fingers ex/flex												
MCP	r.											
MCP	l.											
PIP/IP	r.											
PIP/IP	l.											
DIP	r.											
DIP	l.											
Power grip – distance fingertip-palm	r.											
	l.											
Hook grip	r.											
	l.											
Thumb abduction		r.		l.				r.		l.		
Opposition		r.		l.				r.		l.		
Peg board		r. sec.		l.				r. sec.		l.		
Pain												
Sensibility												
Other (blisters, scars, trophic changes)												

8.7.2 Assessment Form for the Hand – Range of Motion/Sensibility/Pain/Grip forms/Dexterity

The assessment of the range of motion using the AO neutral-0 method is complicated when there are deformities in DEB. It requires a great deal of time and shows little relevance to daily life. The following assessment form has therefore been based on an assessment for rheumatology which focused on deformities and contractures of the joints and different grips. It can provide better information about management of daily life (cf. Harrweg 2006).

ASSESSMENT FORM – HAND
Range of motion/sensibility/pain/grip forms/dexterity

Patient:		Date of birth:	
Date:		Tel.:	
Diagnosis:			
Date of surgery:		Therapist:	
School/profession:		Doctor:	
Dominance: ☐ right ☐ left			
Special notes:			
Aims of intervention:			

Left	INSPECTION	Right
☐	State of the tissue (colour, trophic changes)	☐
☐	Blisters (where?)	☐
☐	Scars (where?)	☐
☐	Muscle atrophy (where?)	☐
☐	Hyperkeratosis	☐
	Contractures/pattern of contractures	
	Wrist	
☐	Flexion contracture	☐
☐	Ulnar deviation	☐

Left	Transverse arch	Right
☐	In order	☐
☐	Flattened	☐
	MCP joints II–V	
☐	Ulnar deviation	☐
☐	Webbing	☐
☐	Flexion contracture	☐
☐	Extension contracture	☐
	MCP joint I	
☐	Hyperextension	☐
☐	Webbing	☐
	PIP and DIP joints II–V	
☐	Extension deficit PIP	☐
☐	Extension deficit DIP	☐
☐	Flexion deficit PIP	☐
☐	Flexion deficit DIP	☐
	Thumb	
☐	Adduction position	☐
☐	Pseudo-opposition position	☐
	Other abnormality	
☐	Shortened fingers (bone reabsorption)	☐
	SENSIBILITY	
☐	Hypersensibility (where?)	☐
☐	Hyposensibility (where?)	☐
	PAIN	
☐	Where exactly?	☐
	What does it feel like?	
	When?	
☐	At rest	☐
☐	Movement	☐

Left		Right
☐	Taking strain	☐
☐	Pressure pain (where?)	☐
	FUNCTION	
	Opening of the hand	
☐	In order	☐
☐	Restricted	☐
☐	Not possible	☐
	Power grip	
☐	In order	☐
☐	Restricted	☐
☐	Not possible	☐
	Hook grip	
☐	In order	☐
☐	Restricted	☐
☐	Not possible	☐
	Abduction DII–DV	
☐	In order	☐
☐	Restricted	☐
☐	Not possible	☐
	Radial abduction of the thumb	
☐	In order	☐
☐	Restricted	☐
☐	Not possible	☐
	Opposition of the thumb	
	Hold objects	
☐	Big	☐
☐	Medium	☐
☐	Small	☐

Left	Range of motion of the wrist	Right
	Radial	
☐	In order	☐
☐	Restricted	☐
☐	Not possible	☐
	Ulnar	
☐	In order	☐
☐	Restricted	☐
☐	Not possible	☐
	Dorsal	
☐	In order	☐
☐	Restricted	☐
☐	Not possible	☐
	Palmar	
☐	In order	☐
☐	Restricted	☐
☐	Not possible	☐
	FUNCTIONAL PHASE OF THE DEFORMITIES	
	Power grip	
☐	Normal	☐
☐	Restricted	☐
☐	Not possible	☐
	Precision grips	
☐	Two-point precision grip	☐
☐	Three-point precision grip	☐
☐	Key grip	☐
☐	Interdigital grip	☐
	Dexterity	
	Moberg pickup test	
	Compensation	
	Possibilities	

The grip strength is not measured because this puts strain on the hand; a full, firm power grip can also cause pressure on the skin which may cause injury, and this should be avoided.

8.7.3 Assessment Form for the Hand – Longitudinal Growth and Pseudosyndactyly

The hand is placed on a piece of paper with the fingers in full extension and spread out, and the contour is drawn. On this drawing the axes of the fingers from capitatum to the fingertips are marked. Then the distance between capitatum and the interdigital space is marked. The result is then dated and the process is repeated each year so that the results can be compared. To ensure that the measurement is as exact as possible, the fingers should be abducted from each other as far as possible and the position of capitatum carefully marked. This method can only be used when there are hardly any contractures.

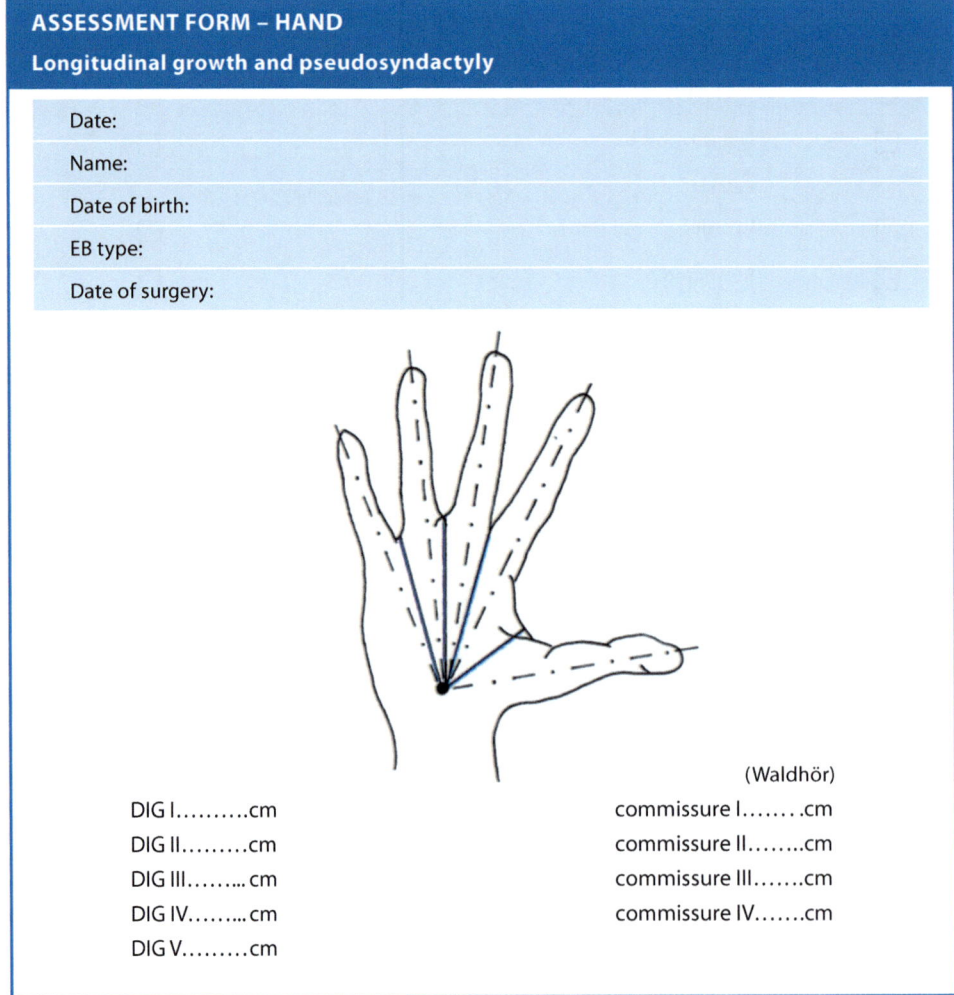

ASSESSMENT FORM – HAND
Longitudinal growth and pseudosyndactyly

Date:

Name:

Date of birth:

EB type:

Date of surgery:

(Waldhör)

DIG I..........cm   commissure I........cm
DIG II.........cm   commissure II........cm
DIG III.........cm   commissure III.......cm
DIG IV.........cm   commissure IV.......cm
DIG V.........cm

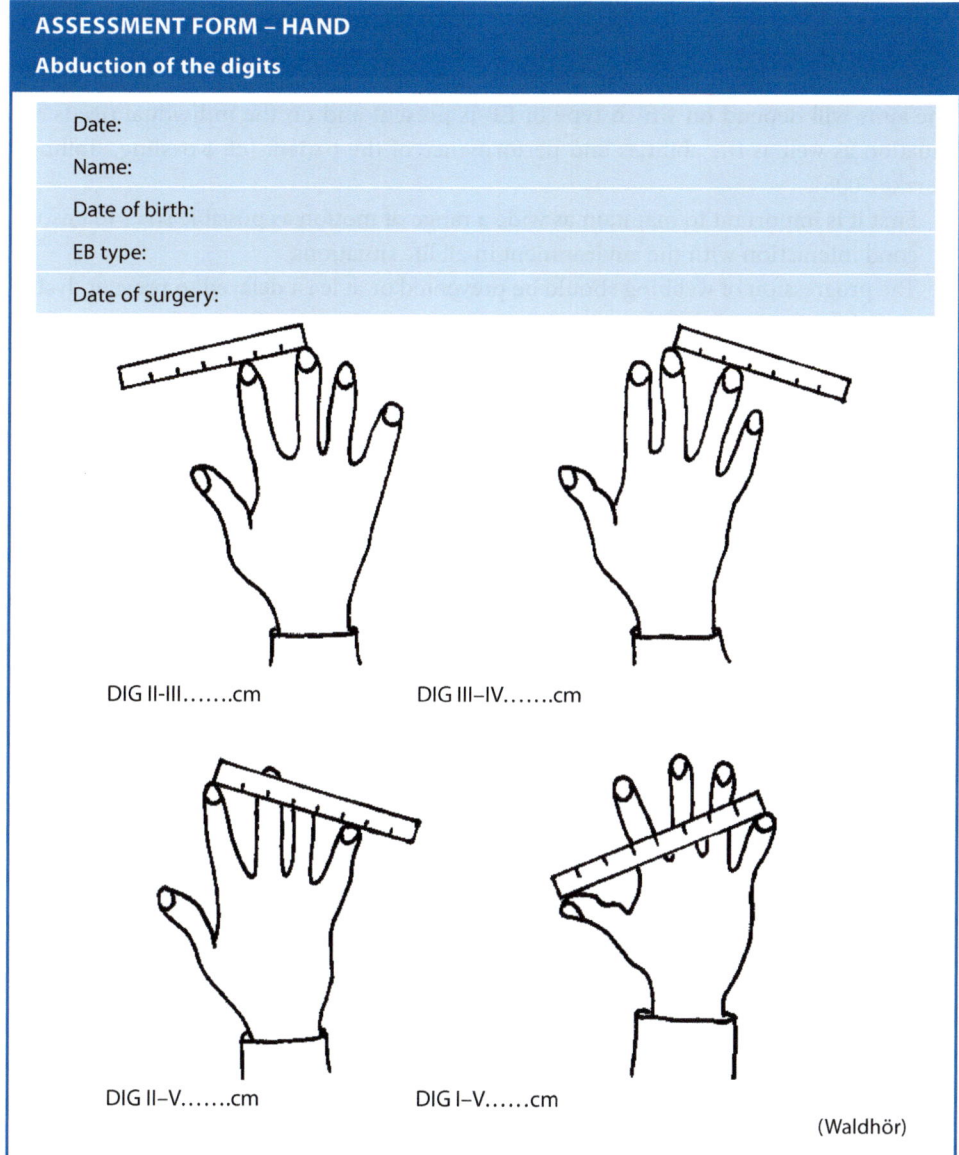

ASSESSMENT FORM – HAND

Abduction of the digits

Date:

Name:

Date of birth:

EB type:

Date of surgery:

DIG II-III.......cm   DIG III–IV.......cm

DIG II–V.......cm   DIG I–V......cm

(Waldhör)

8.7.4   Assessment Form for the Hand – Abduction of the Digits

This form is mainly used for adults who only have webbing without any flexion contracture. It cannot be used during growth because the length and the abduction of the fingers correlate with each other.

The abduction of the fingers can be measured from the tip of the middle finger to the fingers on either side. The distance between the index finger and the little finger can also be measured. The distance between the thumb and the little finger gives the full spread of the hand.

8.8   Occupational Therapy

8.8.1   Aims of Intervention

The aims will depend on which type of EB is present and on the individual needs and situation as well as the abilities and performance of the patient (cf. Koesling, Bollinger Herzka 2008).

- First it is important to maintain as wide a range of motion as possible so as to ensure good interaction with the environment in all life situations.
- The progression of webbing should be prevented or at least delayed to prevent dystrophy of the intrinsic muscles.
- Restrictions due to painful blistering should be prevented.
- Protective and relieving postures should be prevented.

8.8.2   Bandaging and Compression Gloves

To prevent the development of adhesions, the interdigital spaces can be bandaged (see Fig. 8.17a).

As an alternative to bandaging in order to prevent webbing, compression gloves may be considered, but with reservations. The skin must be able to tolerate the pulling on and off of the gloves. There is a zip on the back of the hand, and the gloves have a certain pressure so as to be effective. They encompass each proximal phalanx but should not hinder the dexterity of the fingers in any way. A pad in the palm should maintain the thenar eminence in abduction and limit the adduction of the thumb and the

to some degree so as to maintain the opening of the first commissure (web space) as long as possible (see Fig. 8.17b).

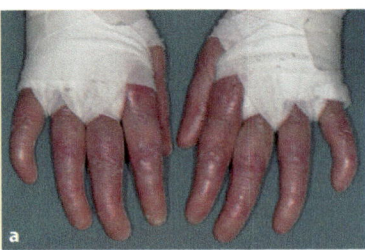 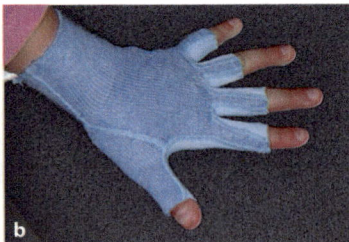

○ **Fig. 8.17 a** Bandaging the interdigital spaces (Hametner). **b** Compression glove (Hametner)

8.8.3   Splinting for Contracture Prophylaxis

Night resting splints are the most effective measure to provide the patient with full freedom of movement during the day, while at night they are worn alternatively on the right and left hand to counteract the flexion contracture.

In splinting there is a wide variety of possibilities which have shown varyingly good results in practice. Pölzleitner (2007) used a parental questionnaire for her thesis to evaluate which models had been successful and which not and what problems and difficulties had arisen. The following information is largely based on these results.

Apart from night resting splints the use of extension stretch splints, which were worn during the day, was tried out. This type of splinting did, however, not prove itself in practice.

Principles of Splinting

The general splinting principles, such as the three-point principle and resting in an immobilised position against the development of deformities, are used. Adhering to these criteria should prevent or correct malpositions and maintain the function of the hands as long as possible. Preventing and minimising contractures is the aim.

Splinting should begin at the first signs of contractures of the fingers. It is advisable to wear anti-webbing bandaging in the splint. They are the most effective measure to delay the development of pseudosyndactyly. Splints with this aim are not as effective as bandaging.

Splints should be kept as simple as possible, but at the same time they must be chosen to have the maximum effect possible. They should be lined with a soft padding or allow gauze to be placed inside; this is more hygienic than a fixed lining because it can be changed daily. The edges of a splint often present a danger of injury; a soft lining is often not enough to overcome this. Sometimes it is necessary to bandage over the complete splint or to pull a mitten over it. Splints should be worn alternatively right and left, not both at the same time. Changes in the range of motion of the fingers or wrist indicate that the splint needs to be refitted. It is important that the splint is positioned exactly right so that it causes no pressure or pain.

The handling of the splint is also very important. Parents will usually put the splint onto children, but for adolescents it is crucial that they can manage this for themselves. This must therefore be practiced and checked in therapy. It is important that the splint be aesthetically acceptable to the wearer in order to have a positive influence on the compliance.

Positioning the Joints

One alternative is to position the joints in extension and abduction:
- Wrist
  - Sagittal plane: the 0 position when the wrist has full movement and no danger of contractures, 20–30° extension when there is a danger of contractures developing
  - Frontal plane: the axis should be straight
- Hand (metacarpus) – maintain or form the transverse arch of the MCP joints
- Fingers – extension in all joints with a slight abduction and central axis
- Thumb – extension in all joints with the largest possible radial abduction to work against an adduction and pseudo-opposition contracture (see Fig. 8.8a,b). It is important to ensure that there is no compensatory hyperextension because of an adduction contracture in the MC I joint.

This type of splint is required when there are contractures which lead to a fist (see Fig. 8.5a,b) and contractures of the MCP joints in the lumbrical position (see Fig. 8.7a,b).

A further possibility is the lumbrical or intrinsic-plus position:

- Wrist
  - Sagittal plane: 30° extension
  - Frontal plane: the axis should be straight
- Hand (metacarpus) – maintain or form the transverse arch of the MCP joints – MCP joints 60–80° flexion
- Fingers – PIP and DIP joints in extension with a slight abduction and central axis
- Thumb – extension in all joints with the largest possible radial abduction to work against an adduction and pseudo-opposition contracture. It is important to ensure that there is no compensatory hyperextension because of an adduction contracture in the MC I joint.

This type of splint is required when there are contractures of the PIP joints (see Fig. 8.3a,b) or contractures of both finger joints (PIP and DIP), which may develop into a hook grip (see Fig. 8.4a,b).

Splinting must be individually fitted according to the contracture pattern and the individual contracture of each finger or joint; this includes not only the choice of splint, but also the placement of the straps.

8.8.4 Types of Splint for Contracture Prophylaxis

Splints Made out of Soft Putty Elastomer (see Fig. 8.18)
This type of contracture prophylaxis can be used with relatively small children, where the time taken to fit a thermoplastic splint makes the compliance more difficult. Soft putty elastomer makes it easier to work quickly, and the child only needs to concentrate on the procedure for a short time. It is not possible to correct the position of the wrist with this method.

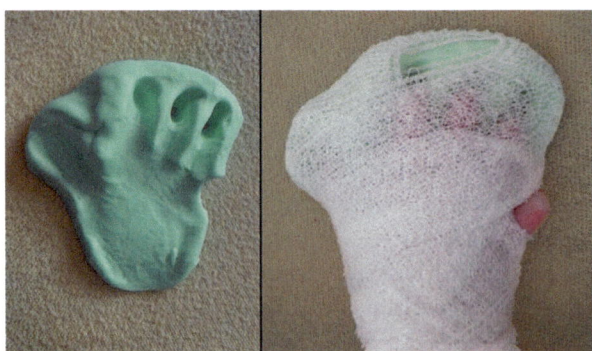

■ **Fig. 8.18** Splints made of soft putty elastomer

Night Resting Splint (see Fig. 8.19a,b)
The night resting splint must be fitted so as to provide the best possible correction of the extension deficit of the fingers and the radial abduction deficit of the thumb.

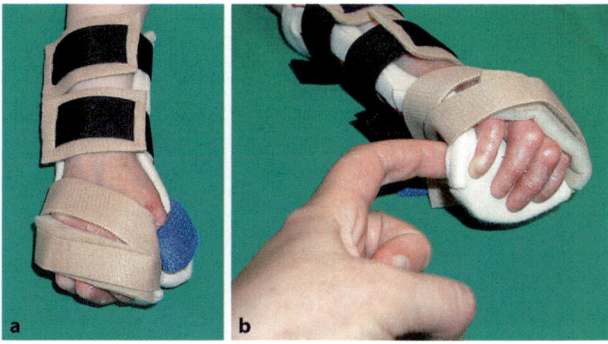

🔹 **Fig. 8.19 a** Night resting splint against PIP contractures. **b** PIP contractures of almost 90°

The splint has the advantage of easy handling and that any necessary bandages on the hand or single fingers can be worn easily at the same time. It can also be refitted to new situations at any time.

Night Resting Splint with Separate Fingers (see Fig. 8.20)
With this variation of the palmar night resting splint the fingers are each held separately with Velcro straps.

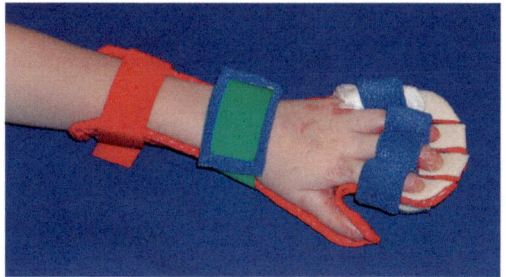

🔹 **Fig. 8.20** Night resting splint with separate fingers

This splint has the advantage that the force on each finger can be individually regulated and the position of the pressure can be exactly placed. The fingers are placed slightly in abduction through the positioning of the straps. A disadvantage is that only bandages of a specific thickness can be worn. The handling is also more complicated than the splint shown in Fig. 8.19, and it cannot be recommended for very small hands.

Night Resting Splint with Silicone Elastomer Inlay (see Fig. 8.21)
Separating and positioning of the fingers is done here with the use of a silicone elastomer inlay.

The handling of this splint is relatively simple and the silicone elastomer inlay can be reformed at any time.

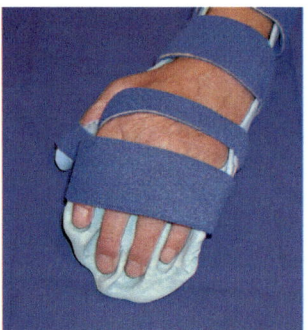

■ **Fig. 8.21** Night resting splint with silicone elastomer inlay

This type of splinting is popular with many patients, but for others the silicone elastomer inlay is too hard and rigid. Bandages can hardly be placed in variable positions, because the impression is that made at the time the inlay is formed.

8.8.5 Exercises to Prevent Deformities

It is important to consider children within their own environment. It is necessary to integrate the parents, grandparents, brothers and sisters, teachers and any other persons important to the child, into the situation.

Therapy offers the possibility of discovering hidden resources and potentials of the child and to give the child support in a new way because sometimes it has come to accept the daily routine without question (cf. Koesling, Bollinger Herzka 2008).

Exercises to prevent deformities are firstly orientated to maintaining the range of motion in the wrist and to exercise the extension and abduction of the fingers.

The programme must naturally be geared towards the age of the child. With toddlers and pre-schoolchildren finger plays and games are recommended (see Figs. 8.22–8.26).

Following are some suggestions out of a large number, which use the fingers in a playful way:

Finger Rhyme 'Here is the Church'

Here is the church,	*Fold hands together so that fingers are hidden inside, with thumbs pressed together and pointing straight up.*
And here is the steeple,	*Raise index fingers and put tips together to form a tall triangle.*
Open the doors	*Separate thumbs.*
And here are the people.	*Turn figure 'inside out', to reveal ten fingers interlaced and wriggling.*
Here is the priest	*Place hands back to back.*
Climbing upstairs,	*Link the fingers of the two hands starting with the little fingers.*
And here he is Saying his prayers.	*Twist hands round so that the thumb of one hand is surrounded by the fingers of the other hand.*

Finger Rhyme 'I Have Ten Fingers'

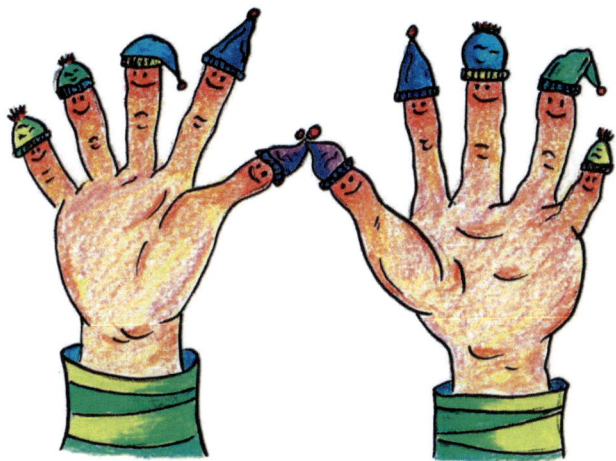

◘ **Fig. 8.22** Finger puppets (Waldhör)

» I have ten fingers   *hold up both hands, fingers spread*
  And they all belong to me,   *point to self*
  I can make them do things-
  Would you like to see?

» I can shut them up tight   *make fists*
  I can open them wide   *open hands*
  I can put them together   *place palms together*
  I can make them all hide   *put hands behind back*

» I can make them jump high   *hands over head*
  I can make them jump low   *touch floor*
  I can fold them up quietly   *fold hands in lap*
  And hold them just so.

Bell Glove for Finger Games

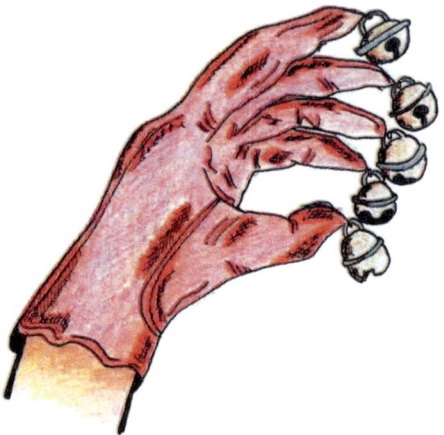

◉ **Fig. 8.23** Glove with bells (Waldhör)

Finger Rhyme 'This is the Way we Wash our Hands'

Make the relative actions

» This is the way we wash our hands,
  Wash our hands, wash our hands.
  This is the way we wash our hands
  So early in the morning.

Substitute:

» ... Brush our teeth
  ... Comb our hair
  ... Give a hug, etc.

'This is the Way to Build a House'
(Sing to the tune of 'Here we come gathering nuts in May' or 'This is the way we wash our hands'.)

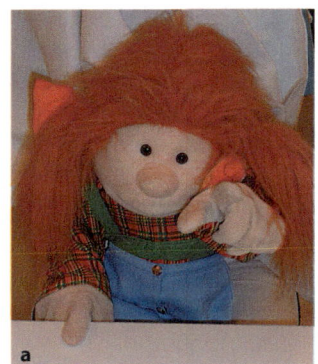

» This is the way to build a house, build a house, build a house.
This is the way to build a house each and every day.

Tap alternatively with the index fingers on the table.

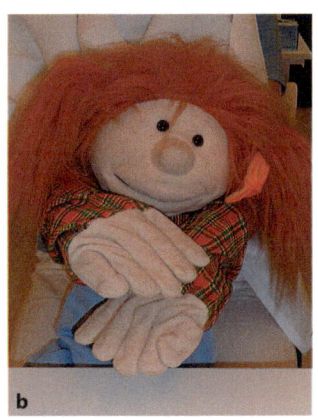

» This is the way to put up the walls, put up the walls, put up the walls.
This is the way to put up the walls with sturdy 2 × 4s (two by fours).

Hands alternate over each other.

» Now we need the windows and doors, windows and doors, windows and doors.
Now we need the windows and doors to keep us locked in tight.

Index fingers and thumbs form a rectangle.

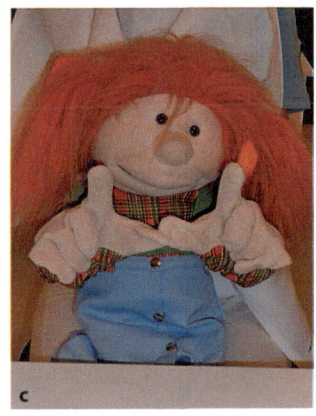

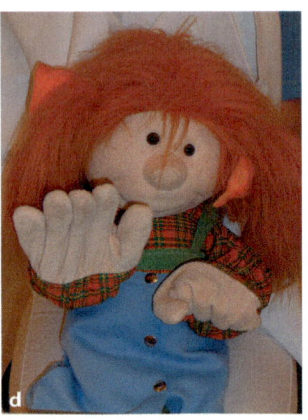

» All we need to do is paint, to do is paint, to do is paint.
All we need to do is paint to make the house look bright.

Imitate painting and rolling.

» This is the way we string the wire, string the wire, string the wire,
This is the way we string the wire, to start the electricity.

Pulling motions with both fists.

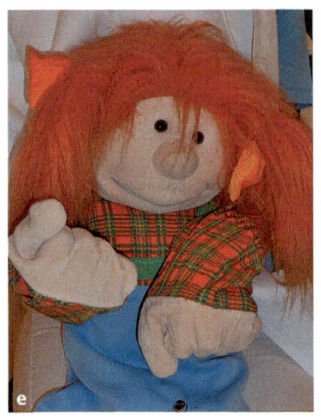

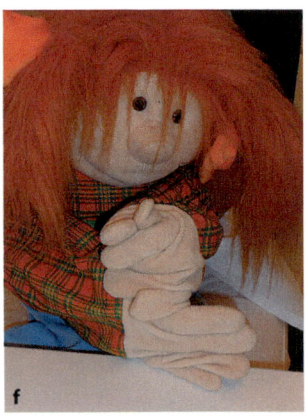

» This is the way the pipe must fit, pipe must fit, pipe must fit.
This is the way the pipe must fit so water can come out.

One fist holds the thumb of the other hand as though pulling.

» Do you see our job is done, job is done, job is done?
Do you see our job is done? Our house is now all built.

Clap hands rhythmically.

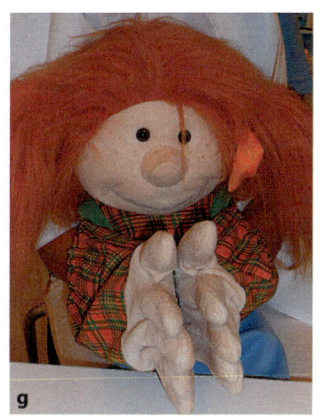

🔲 **Fig. 8.24a–g** Finger rhyme

Finger Rhyme 'Thumbkin'

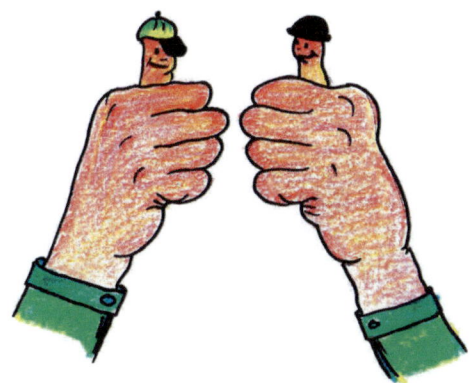

🔲 **Fig. 8.25** Thumbkin (Waldhör)

» Where is Thumbkin?
Where is Thumbkin?
Here I am. Here I am.
How are you this morning?
Very well I thank you.
Run and play. Run and play.

» Where is Pointer?
… Tall Man?
… Ring Man?
… Pinky?
… The whole family?

Finger Rhyme 'Itsy Bitsy Spider'

» Itsy bitsy spider, climbing up the spout,

   'walk' with index and middle fingers up the other arm

» Down came the rain and washed the spider out.

   Both hands wiggle, fingers starting high and 'falling' down

» Out came the sunshine and dried up all the rain,

   Both arms open up a big circle

» Itsy bitsy spider, climbing up the spout again

   'walk' with index and middle fingers up the other arm

Playful Finger Exercises

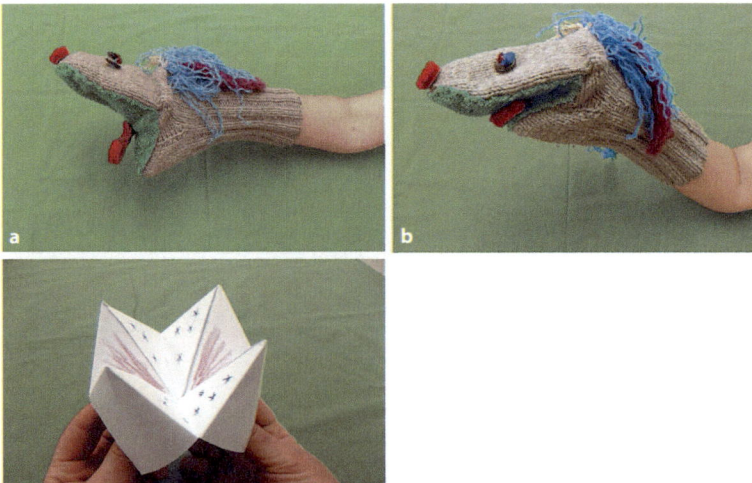

🔲 **Fig. 8.26 a** 'Socky' – Finger extension. **b** 'Socky' – Lumbrical grip. **c** A fortune teller – Finger extension

Hand Massage

When washing or changing bandages, the hands and fingers can be massaged and stretched; stretch the thumbs out and stretch the PIP and DIP joints. This sort of hand massage can also be a way of giving attention to the child. A relationship is built up and the touching of hands can be a pleasant experience. The exercises can also be combined with stories, especially for small children.

Painting on a Mirror

Finger paint or shaving cream painted on a mirror can exercise the fingers and be creative at the same time.

Functional Games

Adolescents and adults will have more fun playing games such as 'Connect Four' or 'Nine Men's Morris'. There are many ways to vary these games: The figures can be held between the fingers so that an extension of the fingers is important (see Fig. 8.27a,b). Other examples are shown in Fig. 8.27c–f.

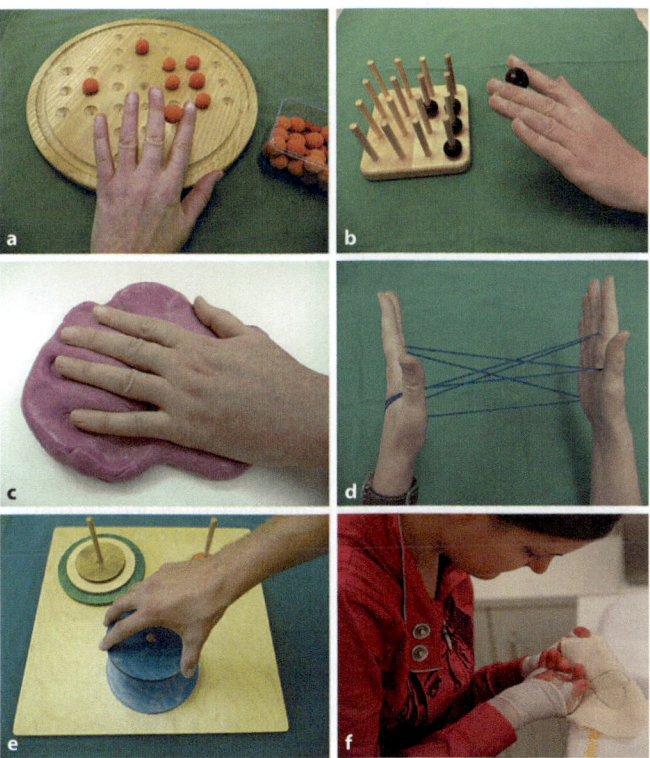

◘ **Fig. 8.27 a** Solitaire. **b** Connect Four. **c** Therapeutic putty. **d** String games. **e** Towers of Hanoi. **f** An affected person using a needle and thread

EXERCISES FOR FINGER EXTENSION AND THUMB ABDUCTION

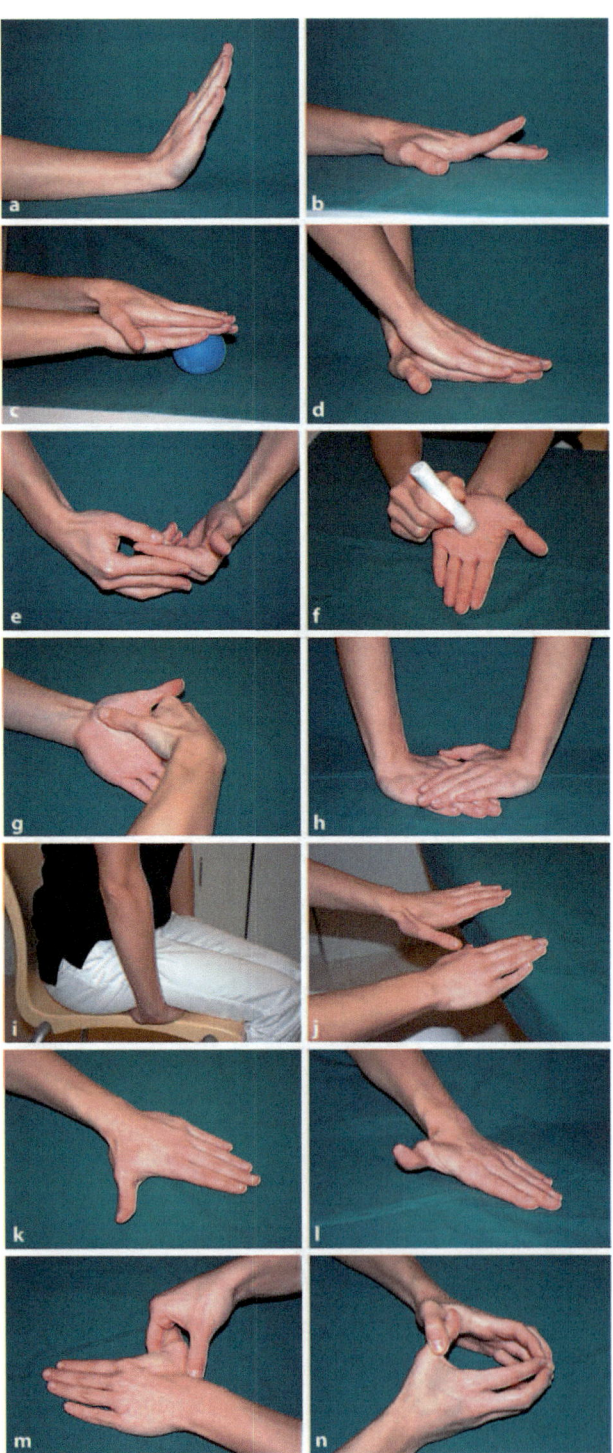

🔲 **Fig. 8.28** **a** Finger and wrist extension. **b** Finger extension of each finger. **c** Stretching the flexor side with a ball. **d** Hands over each other and stroking of the fingers. **e** Stretching the PIP joints. **f** Massage of the hand muscles with a mini-massager relaxes the muscles. **g** Stroking the thenar eminence towards the radial side. **h** Stretching fingers and wrist. **i** Stretching the fingers and wrist (Matschi). **j** Stretching the fingers on a table. **k** Radial abduction of the thumb. **l** Abduction and extension of the thumb. **m** Self-mobilisation: radial abduction of the thumb. **n** Self-mobilisation: palmar abduction of the thumb

8.9 Postoperative Occupational Therapy after Digital Separation

8.9.1 Aims of Treatment

The aims of treatment will depend on the degree of surgery and on how many such operations have been performed. Postoperative treatment brings success by helping to reduce the severity of limitation of hand function, with the obvious restrictions on independence and by enabling the achievement of activities important to the client. The first aim is to influence the process of disablement positively.

The aims of treatment in general:
- Maintain or recover the range of motion of all joints which are not affected by bone fusion.
- Desensitise hypersensitive areas to enable fine motor dexterity.
- Enable the gliding of tendons.
- Reduce contractures and scarring which limit movement.
- Enable grasp (two- and three-point precision grip, interdigital grip …).
- Enable the best possible conditions for ADLs.
- Enable participation in all the different areas of life such as school, profession, leisure and sport.
- Provide everything which the patient needs to maintain his or her quality of life.

8.9.2 Postoperative Splinting

Eating Device

The kind of splint needed for eating depends on the time at which it is introduced after the operation.

If both hands are operated on at the same time, then using an eating device which can be worn over plaster and bandaging maintains independence at mealtimes (see Fig. 8.29).

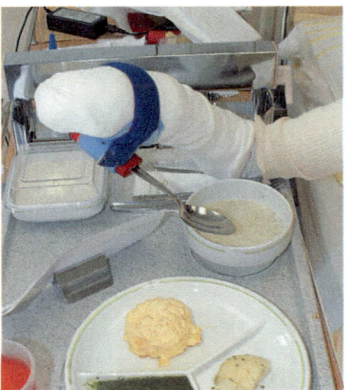

◘ Fig. 8.29 Eating device made of splinting material (Hametner)

Postoperatively, there are often some remaining deformities, depending on how long the fingers were joined, on the degree of preoperative deformity and on the number of previous operations. Apart from flexion contractures of the fingers, which cannot be completely corrected, there is often a tendency for the MCP joints to show ulnar deviation.

A further fundamental point is how far the fingers could be stretched intra-operatively and what positions the axes of the fingers have while they are immobilised in plaster during the healing of the largest incisions. If the fingers have been spread out wide and the MCP joints left in hyperextension to help delay the further development of deformities, this can lead to an unphysiological position of the joints. The functional axes of the fingers can be reduced, but this encourages ulnar deviation; on a long-term basis, there is a danger of subluxation of the MCP joints (see Fig. 8.30).

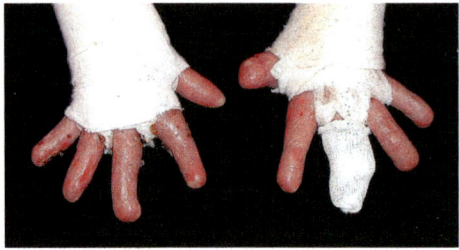

Fig. 8.30 Unphysiological finger axes (Hametner)

The postoperative splinting is similar to the splinting for contracture prophylaxis (see Chap. 8.8.3). The type of splint chosen will depend on the preoperative contractures.

In the case of a lumbrical position in the splint, care must be taken because pressure in the palm of the hand around the MCP joints may interfere with the healing process. In this case it is advisable to fit a splint in the lumbrical position only after the wounds have fully healed.

The aim of splinting is to work as far as possible against the individual deformities and to solve the specific problems. An effort is made to treat the extension of each digit according to its needs; this means that the splint must be made and adjusted to each individual digit.

Dorsal Splint with Palmar Cover

This type has proved to be the best thermoplastic splint for the care of the hands while the operation wounds are healing (see Fig. 8.31a–c).

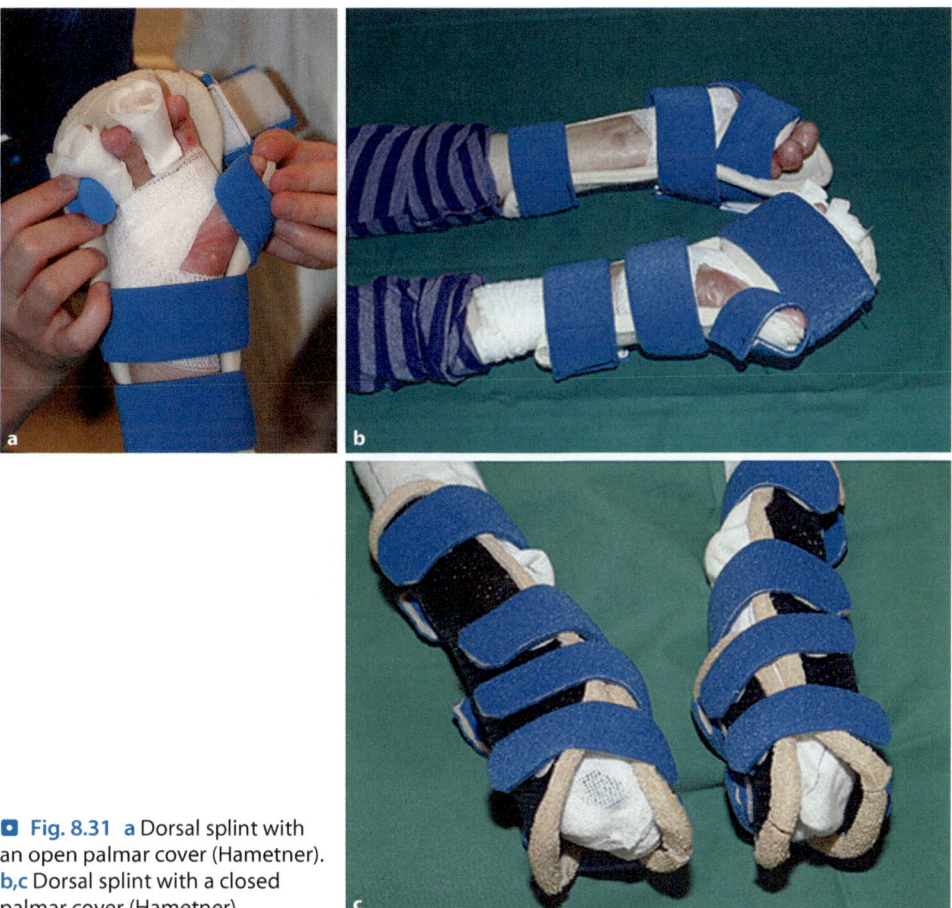

◨ **Fig. 8.31 a** Dorsal splint with an open palmar cover (Hametner). **b,c** Dorsal splint with a closed palmar cover (Hametner)

The cover of this splint can be loosened to relieve pain, to move the finger or to allow air onto the wounds to help the healing process. Bandage thickness will vary pursuant to needs; it is easy to fit the splint accordingly.

Dorsal Splint with Loops for the Individual Fingers

This splint is provided only after the wounds have healed. Each finger is placed in a loop similarly to a dynamic splint. The loops must be placed as distally as possible, and they are attached with a firm cord which can be tightened or loosened and fixed with Velcro to the dorsal side of the splint.

The aim is to regulate each finger so as to give consideration to the different ranges of motion of the individual fingers. At the same time, it allows for individual loosening to relieve the pain of sores (see Fig. 8.32 a–c).

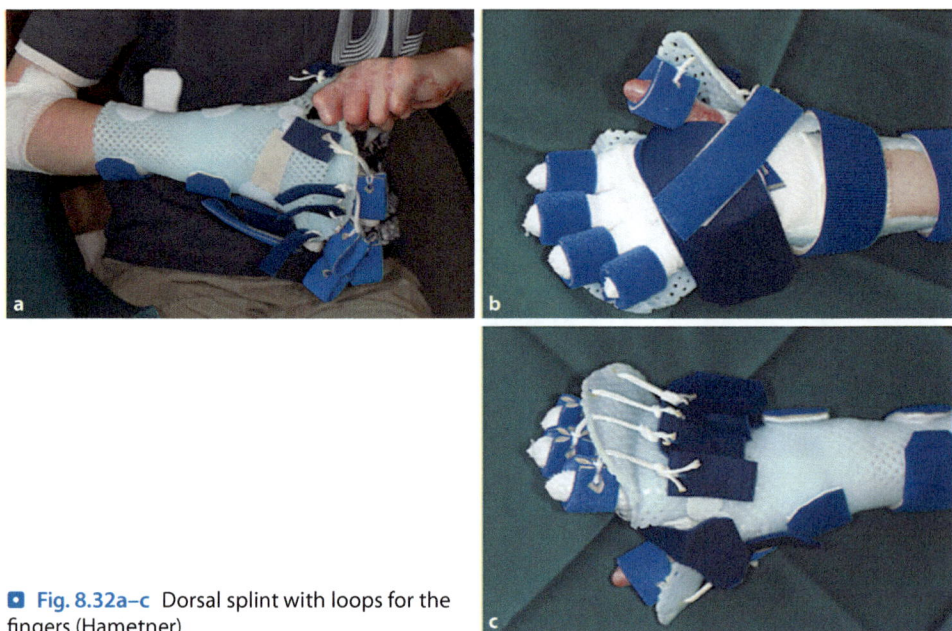

Fig. 8.32a–c Dorsal splint with loops for the fingers (Hametner)

Palmar Splint to Correct Deformities

This splint aims to correct deformities, especially the ulnar deviation of the fingers, in that the straps pull the fingers radially and the hand (metacarpals) towards ulnar. In this way, the ulnar deviation and secondary tendon luxation of extensor digitorum communis are opposed (see Fig. 8.33a–d).

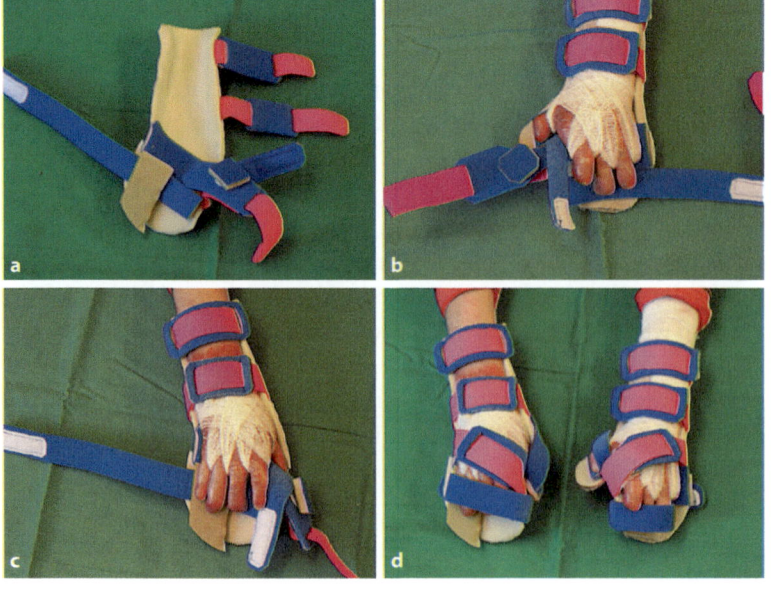

Fig. 8.33
a Palmar splint left (Hametner).
b Palmar splint with finger correction left (Hametner). **c** Palmar splint with finger correction right (Hametner).
d Palmar splints with finger correction (Hametner)

Palmar Splint to Correct the Fingers Individually

This splint aims to solve the individual problems of each finger (see Fig. 8.34a,b).

The fitting of this splint can be complicated. The straps can be difficult to manage, and so the instructions to the parents are extremely important.

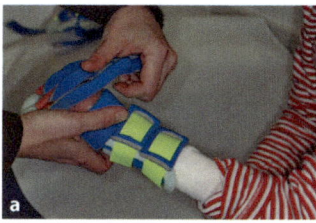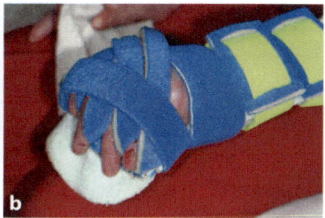

☑ **Fig. 8.34a,b** Correction of ulnar deviation in the MCP joints (Hametner)

8.9.3   Postoperative Problems

Clinical observation over a number of years shows that, with an increasing number of operations, the skin becomes more and more hypersensitive. Some fingers can become so sensitive to touch that the ability to tolerate a splint diminishes and it becomes more difficult to use this treatment. Ludwikowski (2009) described the shortening of the nerve and blood vessel sheaths and the resulting numbness of the finger, for example when force from the splint is exerted on it because the finger is pulled into flexion during the night. The fingertips can become white; the blood flow is insufficient. Because of the way the contractures continue to develop, repeated operations in the same area are necessary, e.g. in the MCP area of the little finger, the PIP joints or the first interdigital space. The operations sometimes have to be repeated within 1–3 years. This fact also has an effect on the scarring, state of the tissue, sensitivity and blood flow.

The result of surgery is dependent on a number of factors: the sub-type of the condition, the severity of the contractures, the number of operations, the type of splinting and, last but not least, the compliance and stamina of the client.

8.9.4   Assessment Form for the Hand – Sensibility

The following form is designed to document changes of sensitivity resulting from operations. It shows the quality of sensation and the distribution in the different zones of the palm of the hand in a clear way. As there is no primary nerve injury, but rather a disturbance of the nerve conduction because of the pressure from scars or small lesions of the nerves of the fingers or from trophic changes, it is useful to have a descriptive record of the quality of the sensation.

It is of course also possible to use the standardised two-point discrimination test or the Semmes–Weinstein filament test.

System for assessing sensation:

- Anaesthesia: No awareness of a stimulus in the region is present.
- Hypoaesthesia: A stimulus is perceived in the region but not as strongly as on the non-affected side. This is a sign of a partial interruption of the neural conduction.
- Hyperaesthesia: A stimulus is perceived more intensively than on the non-affected side. This functional disturbance of the neural conduction happens frequently in cases of reinnervation.
- Paraesthesia: The patient has feelings of 'pins and needles' in the described region although no stimulus is present. This indicates that there is some degree of compression of the nerve.
- Dysaesthesia: A stimulus in the region is perceived wrongly, e.g. a light touch may cause pain or be perceived as hot or cold. These disturbances occur when there has been continual mechanical stimulation of the nerve, e.g. from plaster or a splint or during a process of reinnervation (cf. Koesling, Bollinger Herzka 2008).

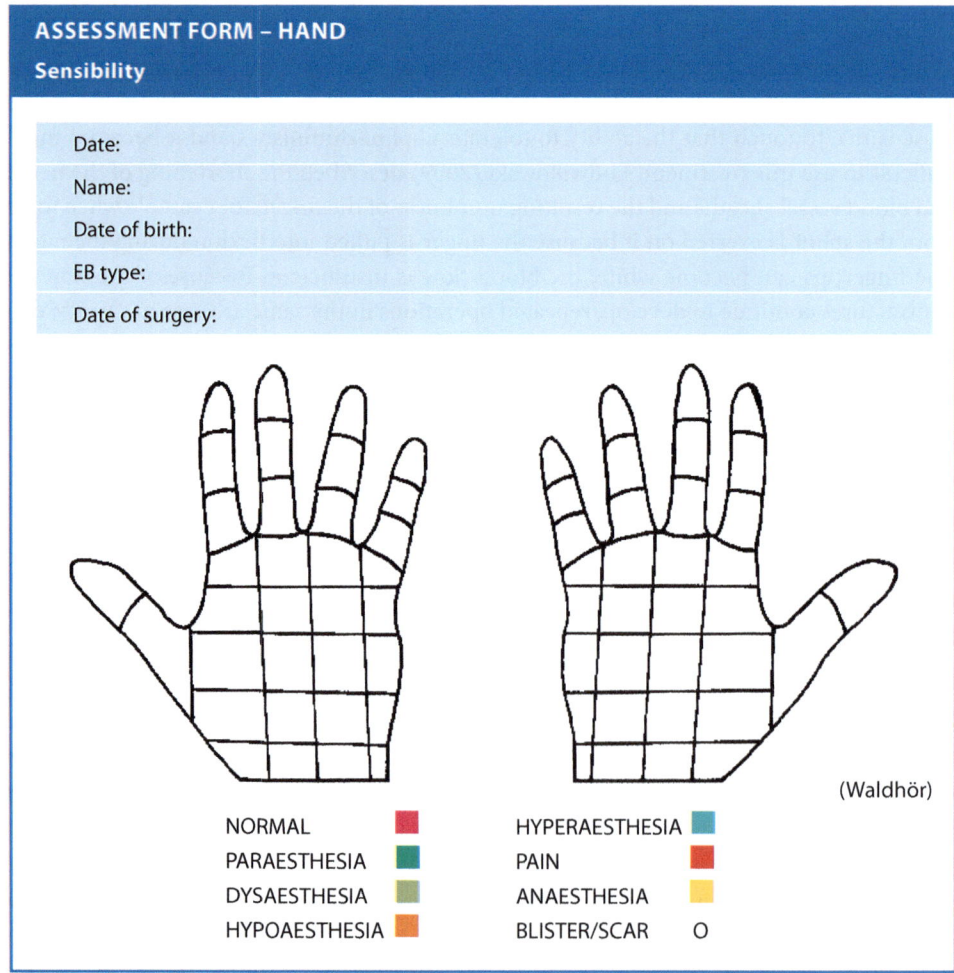

ASSESSMENT FORM – HAND
Sensibility

Date:

Name:

Date of birth:

EB type:

Date of surgery:

(Waldhör)

NORMAL	■	HYPERAESTHESIA	■
PARAESTHESIA	■	PAIN	■
DYSAESTHESIA	■	ANAESTHESIA	■
HYPOAESTHESIA	■	BLISTER/SCAR	O

8.9.5 Training of Sensibility

There are two concepts of sensibility training, desensitisation and reeducation.

In the case of people with EB desensitisation is used more often so it is described here in some detail, while reeducation is given less attention.

Desensitisation

Patients with hypersensitivity overreact to stimuli with pain or unpleasant sensations. The aim of desensitisation is to change the tolerance to the stimuli and so achieve an improved performance in activities of daily life.

Before starting the training, it is necessary to find out which region is most hypersensitive and which less, and to test which stimuli cause the least irritation.

Begin with the region which has the highest tolerance and work towards the more sensitive areas. If that stimulus is no longer unpleasant in the entire affected region, then use the next irritating stimulus.

Suitable materials for this treatment are cotton wool, fur, felt, foam rubber, towelling, Velcro, brushes of varying stiffness, etc.

Sensitivity baths with polystyrene balls, rapeseed, lentils, rice, or ironing beads are only of limited value with EB clients because of the danger of infection. The decision for or against has to be taken individually. A thin throwaway glove could possibly be used for such sensitivity baths.

Apart from the two modalities mentioned, vibration can also be used. This can be done most easily by using a mini-massager. Experience shows that most people with EB find this very pleasant. Different clients react differently, but practice has shown that three to five repetitions of 10 min each, spread over the day, have the best results (Koesling, Bollinger Herzka 2008).

Reeducation

Reeducation aims at changing the structure of perception at a cortical level after nerve injuries. In the early phase of rehabilitation, the concentration is on localising and differentiating between static and moving touch. The rubber on the top of a pencil is moved over the affected area. The patient reports the localisation and in what direction it is moved without being able to see it. Afterwards this is repeated while the patient watches so that the sensation can be associated with what is seen.

Towards the end of the rehabilitation the aim is to recognise the feel of the object and be able to name it. To start with, everyday objects with different shapes, sizes and surfaces are used. The patient learns to differentiate between the objects and to link the new sensation with what had previously been known. The patient should be able to recognise the objects without seeing them. A progression can then be that the shape is the same but the surface is different, or vice versa (cf. Koesling, Bollinger Herzka 2008).

8.9.6 Treatment of Scars

The skin of children is very much influenced by growth. Large scars can cause the problem of the scar tissue growing at only one fifth of the rate of normal skin growth, and so it causes a strong pull (cf. Koesling, Bollinger Herzka 2008). For this reason, treating scars of those in the period of growth is important. After injuries or operations in the hand there is a tendency for the scars to adhere to the tissue below. With wounds over large areas there is a danger of contracture. Scars over joints can significantly affect the range of motion. Hypertrophic scars can cause disturbances to the lymph flow and pain.

The three phases of healing:
1. The inflammatory phase (days 0–5): The phagocytes are present in the wound area as well as cells for the scar formation and resorption. Arterial and venous capillaries and lymphatic vessels all begin to grow.
2. The proliferative phase (days 5–21): Fibroplasia and granulation tissue formation.
3. The remodelling phase (days 21–360): Collagen fibres are rearranged, cross-linked, and aligned along tension lines; the tissue becomes stronger and more elastic.

Treatment of scars can normally begin only once the proliferative phase has started. If it is started too soon, it may extend the inflammatory phase, which should of course be avoided under all circumstances. Skin transplantation can also delay the scar treatment by 1–2 weeks.

Depending on the type of operation, the start of the scar treatment must be decided on according to the case and situation with EB patients. On the whole, the wound healing is slower and so the possibilities of scar treatment need to be tested.

There are different techniques which may be used (see Fig. 8.35).

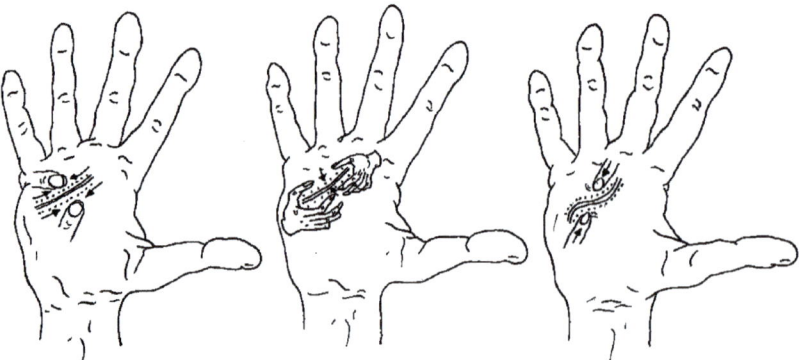

Fig. 8.35 Scar treatment (Waldhör)

Sliding the scar: The thumbs are placed parallel to the scar on either side and the scar is slid over the deeper tissue.

Lifting the skin: The thumbs and index fingers of both hands lift the scar (take extreme care!).
Pushing the scar: The thumbs push along the scar in opposite directions.

Silicone gel or sheeting may also be used. Either a piece covering the scar is bandaged in place or it is used in conjunction with thermoplastic splinting. The continual pressure can have a positive influence on the tissue of hypertrophic scars, contracting wounds and scars after skin transplantations. The blood supply is reduced and the excessive collagen synthesis is decreased (cf. Koesling, Bollinger Herzka 2008).

8.9.7 Treatment of Oedema

After an operation fluid collects in the surrounding tissue. The lack of movement due to the operation results in there being no natural muscle pump, and the fluid does not flow away from the area. Plasma proteins gather in the tissue and adhesions may occur. Cell metabolism is also affected by the increased hydrostatic pressure. The quantity of fluid, the high pressure and the adhesions can lead to a restriction of mobility just when this should become possible again.

Resting
The entire arm should be placed in an elevated position, if possible, above the heart.

Exercises and Muscle Pump
The natural muscle pump can activate the drainage of lymph from the extremity. Opening and closing the hand as far as possible, depending on joint stiffness, should be performed above the head. This reduces the oedema on the back of the hand through the action of the intrinsic muscles.

Manual Lymph Drainage
This gentle stroking process should be something that many EB patients can tolerate.
    First the vessels from the central lymph nodes and lymph vessels are opened through flat circular strokes, and then the fluid is drained from distal to proximal with long flat strokes (cf. Koesling, Bollinger Herzka 2008).

8.9.8 Manual Therapy

It is not always possible to enlarge the range of motion of joints with a limited range only through active movements. With EB patients those joints with some function often have to compensate for other joints that no longer have their function. For this reason, it is extremely important that the physiological roll-glide movement of a joint is retained or recovered as far and as well as possible and then with exercises the joint mobility retained.

Before starting on manual therapy, it is important to make a thorough assessment of the situation:

- The passive examination of the joint movement allows the therapist to feel the limit of movement and experience which structures, such as ligaments, capsules, muscles and, with EB patients, skin, obstruct further movement.
- The joint play gives the impression of how stable the joint is – stable, hypermobile, hypomobile, unstable.
- The isometric resistance gives the impression of the state of the muscles which move and stabilise the joint being examined.

According to the state of the examined periarticular structures, the appropriate treatment such as passive angular movement, traction, translation or compression can be carried out.

8.9.9 Functional Exercises after Operative Digital Separation

The postoperative exercise programme is a difficult chapter in the treatment of DEB. On the one hand, regaining the greatest possible range of motion is an important goal necessary for fine motor and coordination skills. On the other hand, there is the anxiety that through the improved range of motion, especially in the IP joints, the danger of contractures forming is again increased.

This fact is endorsed by the decision of an adult patient who refused to do any exercises after the operation and was only prepared to move her thumb. She had already had several operations and, in the hope of not needing such a distressful operation again in a few years' time, had chosen this course. After a while, some movement could be observed in her finger joints. Through the activation of the intrinsic muscles she used a lumbrical grip instead of a power grip, and instead of the two-finger pinch grip she used the pincer grip. She claimed that she was able to use these grips adequately in everyday life and was not significantly restricted and a further operation could be postponed.

With this strategy she achieved her own goal; a further future operation will probably be considerably smaller than the previous ones, and so the results of pain, immobilisation, and long and difficult bandage changing, as well as the slow wound healing will be less (see Fig. 8.36a–f).

If the best possible dexterity is required, for example to play a musical instrument or to achieve the best possible participation in everyday life, it is important to examine the X-ray images before starting on an exercise programme. Together with a specialist for physical medicine, it is necessary to decide which joints can be expected to achieve what range of motion on account of their condition. For this reason, the full exercise programme presented here can seldom be carried out. The functional possibilities of the individual joints as seen on the X-rays must be assessed and a suitable selection made, or individual exercises can be modified as required for the ability of the finger joints.

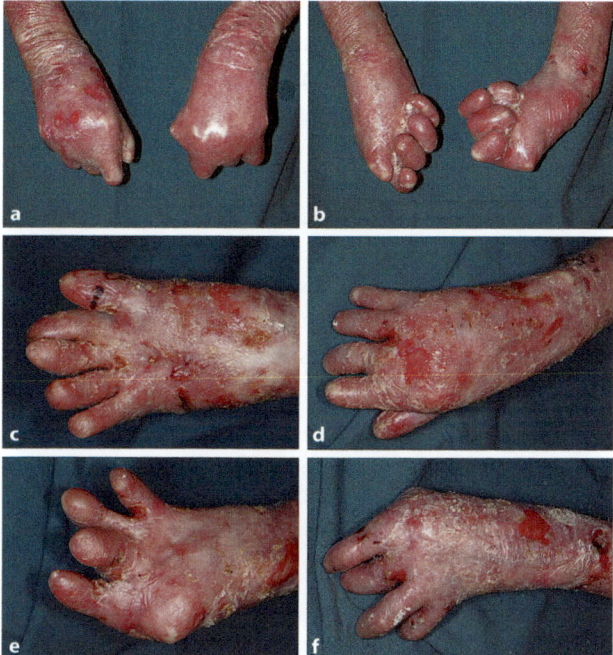

Fig. 8.36 **a** Preoperative status (dorsal) (Hametner). **b** Preoperative contractures and webbing (Hametner). **c** Right hand over 5 years postoperatively (palmar) (Hametner). **d** Right hand over 5 years postoperatively (dorsal) (Hametner). **e** Left hand over 5 years postoperatively (palmar) (Hametner). **f** Left hand over 5 years postoperatively (dorsal) (Hametner)

The longer the adhesions had been present before the operation, the greater the likelihood that the joints are damaged because of the strain on the bones, the lack of use and atrophy of the joint tissues. The degree of the deformity of the joints also depends on how long the adhesions were present. Fusions of the joint surfaces and subluxations can either limit the movement or make it impossible. To achieve the best possible range of motion, the fingers should be wiggled during the change of bandaging as soon as the healing, pain and state of the joints allow it. Abduction and adduction of the fingers and abduction and opposition of the thumb, including the movement of the wrist in all directions, complete the exercises. During this phase, until the wounds have healed completely, splints are worn day and night. They can be opened twice daily for the exercise programme with the bandages in place. Once the healing process is far enough advanced that the hands can be used, it is recommended that night resting splints are worn and exercises for the extension and abduction (see Fig 8.28a–n) and flexion (see Fig. 8.37a–i) are performed.

Experience has shown that it is very difficult to bring back the tendon gliding of the finger flexors (FDP, FDS) because the necessary palmar incisions can lead to adhesions of the tendons very quickly. The two- and three-point pinch grips, which are used a great deal in daily life, require and encourage a gliding of these tendons. The index finger is the one most used and it is therefore usually easiest to regain the movement here, while the movement of the third to fifth fingers deteriorate most. Often it is not possible to regain the flexion in the fourth and fifth fingers. Flexion here is then performed using the lumbrical muscles.

In principle it is easier to regain certain forms of grasp than to retain the extension in the fingers.

The necessity of regular exercising presents a certain barrier. The majority of patients have said in a questionnaire to evaluate the efficacy of OT (Pölzleitner 2007) that they do not do their exercises regularly.

With small children it is best to encourage exercising by using finger rhymes, as recommended above. With adolescents and adults, board games in various sizes and forms can be used as described in the chapter on preventative measures.

POSTOPERATIVE EXERCISES FOR FINGER FLEXION

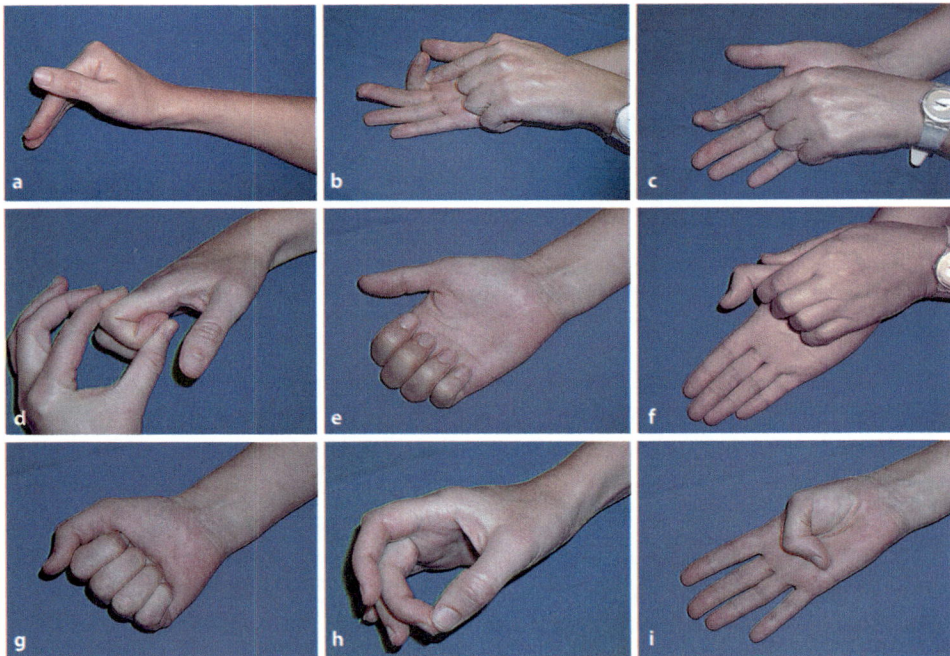

◘ **Fig. 8.37** **a** Lumbrical position. **b** Flexion PIP joint with resistance. **c** Flexion DIP joint with resistance. **d** Hook grip (passive). **e** Hook grip (active). **f** Flexion IP joint of the thumb with resistance. **g** Power grip. **h** Opposition to each fingertip. **i** Maximal thumb opposition with IP flexion

Stretching Exercises

Contractures of the flexor muscles of the forearm develop and the postoperative immobilisation reinforces this. There is an imbalance between the flexors and extensors which can be successfully treated with stretching exercises of the flexors and functional exercises of the antagonists. The most suitable way is to use the 'contract-and-relax' method. Any sort of static stretching can cause too much pressure and force on the neural structures and vessels because of the tissue dystrophy.

- The contract and relax method mentioned above comes from the proprioceptive neuromuscular facilitation (PNF) concept. The wrist is placed in extension; an isometric contraction of the extensor muscles for 5–10 s is done, which then provokes a stretching of those muscles. Following the contraction, the degree of extension is increased, and through a post-isometric blocking a more effective stretching is possible.
- This exercise is repeated from a new starting position two or three times (cf. Koesling, Bollinger Herzka 2008).

FBL Functional Kinetics Klein-Vogelbach

Treatment techniques from FBL Functional Kinetics Klein-Vogelbach (Basel, Switzerland), especially for joint mobilisation, can be used to improve, for example, the pro- and supination as well as for the mobilisation of the finger joints (cf. Koesling, Bollinger Herzka 2008).

Training to Achieve Coordination

To train to achieve coordination, small movement sequences requiring accuracy are repeated, with gradually increasing complexity. A further component is increasing the speed and the fluidity through the automation of the movement.

Dexterity

Dexterity can be obtained by fine motor exercises requiring the coordination of the extrinsic and intrinsic hand muscles. The sensibility, especially of the thumb and the index finger, is necessary for the manipulation of objects. Perception through the receptors of the skin is coordinated with proprioception via the tendons and joints to achieve the fluidity of movement. This explains why sensibility training is vital for the quality of motor activities. For people with EB, desensitisation is very important because the dexterity in many cases is already restricted due to contractures and deformities. One aim can be to work out compensation methods for movements that are impossible (cf. Koesling, Bollinger Herzka 2008).

Cognitive Therapeutic Exercises According to Perfetti

Cognitive therapeutic exercises according to Perfetti can be used in orthopaedics as well as in neurology. The tactile–kinaesthetic stimuli that are recognised help to initiate the planning of movement and the best possible physiological movement.

Stereotypy movements, which develop because of the restrictions and relieving postures, can be interrupted and replaced with more specific movement skills.

Through the improvement of tactile–kinaesthetic perception contracted muscles learn to relax, and there is an improvement in the pain levels (cf. Koesling, Bollinger Herzka 2008).

Feldenkrais Method

Using exercises developed by Moshe Feldenkrais, different variations of movement can be tested and experienced, and it is possible to learn how to move in the most economic manner. In that way, less effort and power is needed and movement can become more accurate. The result is an improved posture and a harmonising of the physical and psychological balance (cf. Koesling, Bollinger Herzka 2008).

Spiraldynamik®

This is a concept for correct anatomical movement based on three dimensions. Complex patterns of movement based on the spiral principle are analysed. It helps to school the perception and coordination of movement in daily life. Swiss doctor Christian Larsen and French physiotherapist Yolande Deswarte laid the foundations for the method (cf. www.spiraldynamik.com, 2012).

8.9.10 Bandaging to Prevent MCP Flexion and Ulnar Deviation

Modified bandaging, as used in chronic polyarthritis, can help to prevent MCP flexion and ulnar deviation (cf. Bitzer, Sörensen 2010).

It also works as an anti-webbing bandage. An effort is made through the pull force of the bandage to influence the position of the fingers in a more radial direction. Care must be taken not to pull the fingers into hyperextension. Using a bandage which sticks to itself is ideal because it has some elasticity, and so it remains possible to bend the MCP joints. The following figures show the individual steps of the bandaging, and its application with a DEB patient (see Fig. 8.38a–j and Fig. 8.39a,b).

BANDAGING

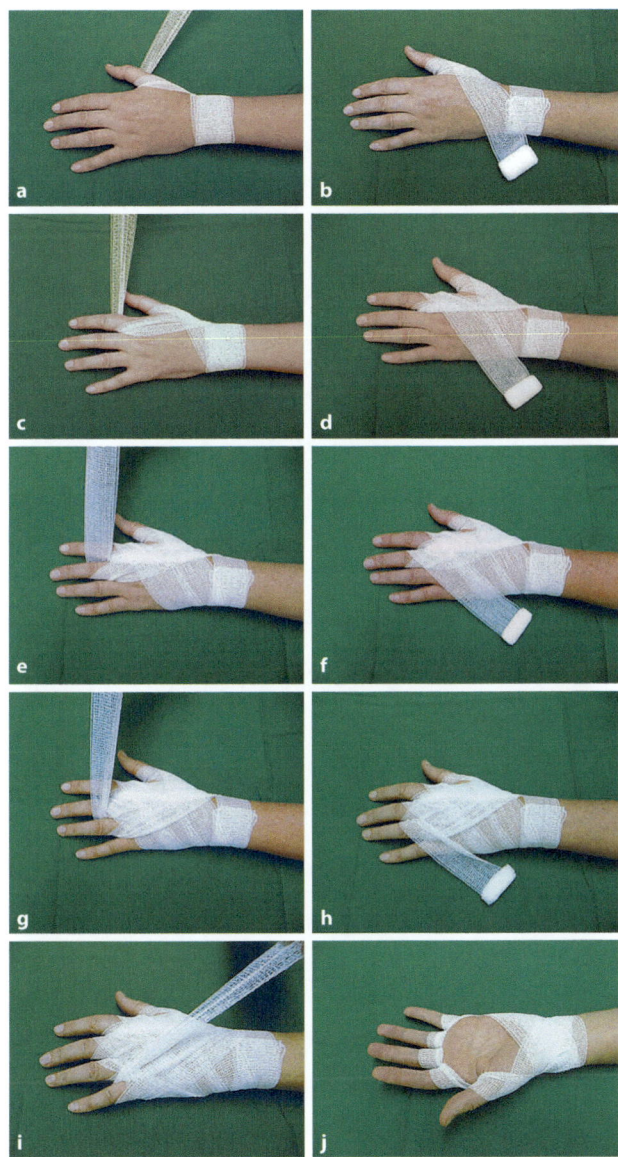

Fig. 8.38a–j Bandaging steps, in alphabetic order

BANDAGING FOR DEB

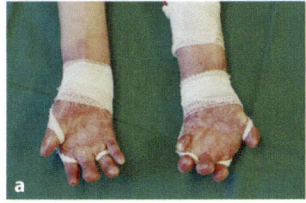

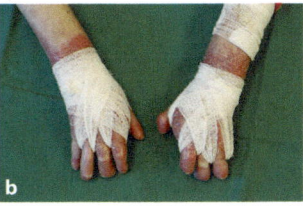

Fig. 8.39 **a** Bandaging for a 15-year-old girl, 1 year postoperatively (palmar) (Hametner). **b** Bandaging for a 15-year-old girl, 1 year postoperatively (dorsal) (Hametner)

9 Rehabilitation of the Foot

Hedwig Weiß

Anatomically, the foot is closely related to the hand, and in some ways the function is also related. It provides the base that carries the whole weight of the body. Posture begins at the feet and rises from there through the other parts of the body.

9.1 The Foot in People with DEB

In the description of the hand in Chap. 8 there was mention of the deformities and skeletal changes of the foot.

The foot gets no relevant therapeutic mention in the few articles about EB that have been published.

Some treatment principles based on the theories of Spiraldynamik® (cf. Larsen 2007; Larsen 2006; Larsen, Miescher, Wickihalter 2007; Lauper 2009) that can be used in intervention with DEB clients are presented here.

The sole of the foot is frequently affected by blistering because of the strain it takes from contact with the ground and shoes while walking. This results in pain, leading to partial weight bearing, either on the lateral side of the foot, on the balls of the feet or on the heels. This has a substantial effect on gait and posture.

The rolling movement of the foot from heel to toe is often painful and may even be impossible due to deformities of the foot. This means that only part of the foot is used, e. g. the forefoot when the heel has blisters and sores, resulting in the development of malpositions of the skeleton of the foot and an imbalance in the coordination of the foot muscles. This poor movement pattern can lead to such secondary complications as contractures in the ankle, knee or hip (see Fig. 9.1).

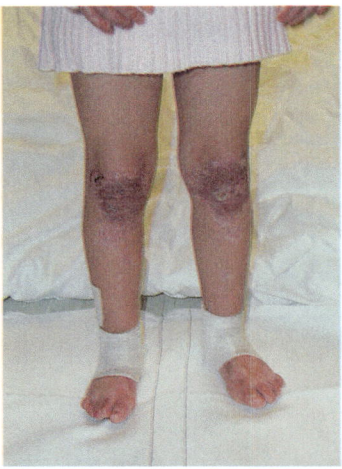

◻ **Fig. 9.1** The feet of an almost-3-year-old child with DEB

9.2 Comparison of Hand and Foot

In pre-humans, the foot and hand were probably very similar. The skeleton of the hand resembles a malleable bone fan with the two horizontal rows of bones at the wrist as a base. The dish-shaped fan consists of five finger rays and has a longitudinal and a transverse arch. The construction allows for stability and precision in fine motor activities (see Fig. 9.2a,b).

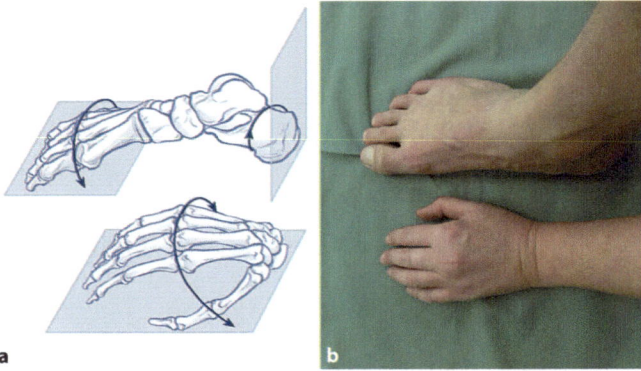

a   b

◘ **Fig. 9.2 a** Comparison of the hand and foot skeleton (© Larsen 2006, p. 5). **b** Arched form of hand and foot

In comparison with the hand, the foot has tarsal bones which are partially vertical to each other; the ankle bone (talus) lies over the huge heel bone (calcaneus). During evolution, a spiral three-dimensional torsion took place which gave the foot weight-bearing stability.

When walking the feet take the entire weight of the body alternately, so that stability and muscle balance are required for taking this load (cf. Köhler, Reber 2006).

9.3 Anatomy and Function of the Foot

9.3.1 The Cuneiform Principle

At the apex of the foot arches there are six wedge-shaped bones: three metatarsals and three tapered cuneiform bones (I–III) that have the same role as the single elements of an architectural arch. This cuneiform principle gives the foot great stability because the cuneiform bones press more and more against each other as the weight increases, so long as the heel takes this weight evenly (see Fig. 9.3).

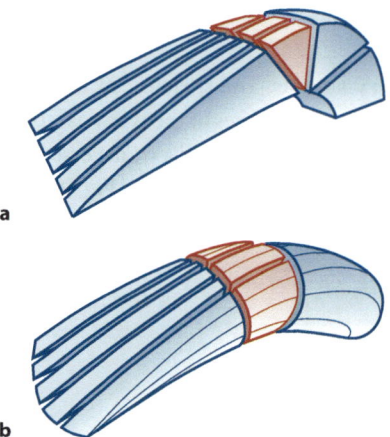

a

b

○ **Fig. 9.3** The cuneiform principle of the skeleton of the foot (© Larsen, Miescher, Wickihalter 2007, p. 32)

9.3.2 The Spiral Principle

The spiralled arch of the foot goes from 'vertical back lateral' to 'horizontal front medial'. This is similar to the wringing out of a cloth, where the hands turn in opposite directions twisting between the two poles. This spiral principle of the foot can be seen when the heel is erect and the MTP joint of the big toe has complete contact with the ground. The arch goes evenly from the outside of the heel to the MTP joint of the big toe – the heel is in eversion (supination) and the forefoot in inversion (pronation) (see Fig. 9.4).

The muscles, ligaments and the connective plantar aponeurosis provide a stability that stretches triangularly from the calcaneus to the MTP joints. The height of the longitudinal arch is held in balance largely by the three muscles tibialis posterior, tibialis anterior and peroneus longus. They are supported by the triceps surae, flexor hallucis longus and flexor digitorum longus. The short muscles of the foot, such as abductor hallucis, flexor hallucis brevis, flexor digitorum brevis and abductor digiti minimi, are also involved (cf. Zukunft-Huber et al. 2011).

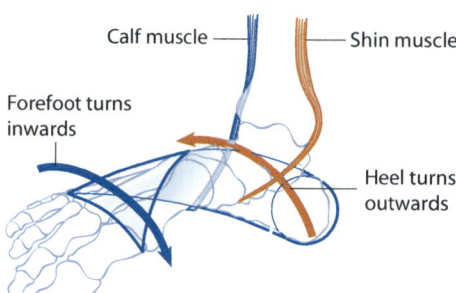

Calf muscle — Shin muscle

Forefoot turns inwards

Heel turns outwards

○ **Fig. 9.4** Spiral principle of the skeleton of the foot (© Larsen, Miescher, Wickihalter 2007, p. 32)

9.3.3 The Transverse Arch

The five joints at the base of the toes form a flat transverse arch, like the letter C. Between them there are dozens of small foot muscles, e.g. interossei pedis, lumbricals, flexor hallucis brevis, adductor hallucis and flexor digiti minimi brevis. These muscles provide for the bending of the MTP joints and the elastic bracing of the forefoot arch. When weight bearing, it is pushed flat on the floor – the muscles between the bones also act as shock absorbers. When rolling the foot from heel to toe in walking, these small muscles are stretched, and then they contract in a reflex manner. This gives the foot forward propulsion while walking. If the shock absorber effect in the forefoot is missing, the knees and hips take a greater strain (see Fig. 9.5).

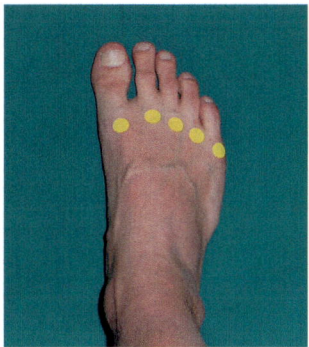

◨ **Fig. 9.5** Forefoot transverse arch

The feet provide a relatively small base when standing. It is however possible for us to organise the body on this small base without losing balance, owing to our differentiated motor adaptation (cf. Nacke 2005).

9.3.4 How DEB Affects these Principles

In DEB the dermatological requirements due to the complications of blistering, sores, adhesions, etc. are dominant over the biomechanical principles. The feet need to take the forces of weight bearing, shearing forces and friction, and so the skin is often in a very bad state and requires bandaging.

Adhesions and webbing of the toes and the impossibility of normal weight bearing on the soles of the feet lead to secondary changes in the skeleton and to muscle atrophy, especially the small muscles which are important for the movement of the toes and the weight shifts during locomotion.

In particular the MTP joint of the big toe may cause problems. It is the impetus for the lift-off movement of each step, and is often unable to take on this function fully because the state of the skin in usually very bad due to the extreme pressure to which this joint is exposed. In addition, contractures in the area of the MTP joints may also play a role.

As with the hands, the toes can become encased in a so-called cocoon (see Fig. 9.6). Spreading out the toes in this situation is impossible, and this leads to an atrophy of the lumbricals and the interossei plantaris and dorsalis.

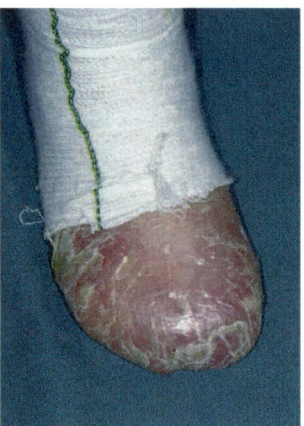

◘ Fig. 9.6 Cocoon-like adhesions

9

9.4 The Pelvis and the Axes of the Legs

9.4.1 The Pelvis

The pelvis is the pivot between the straightened spine and the legs and feet below it. A centred pelvis is the prerequisite for a stable and physiologically correct starting posture for fluid and economic movement. Finding the dynamic centre is an important prerequisite for any activity in an upright position.

To be able to tilt the pelvis into an erect position, the lower back must be relaxed and stretched. The coccyx should be pulled down towards the heels and at the same time the pelvic floor will be activated. The pelvis will tilt up and the hollow back will disappear. The deep abdominal muscles will be activated, while the superficial abdominal muscles and buttocks will remain relaxed (see Fig. 9.7.a,b).

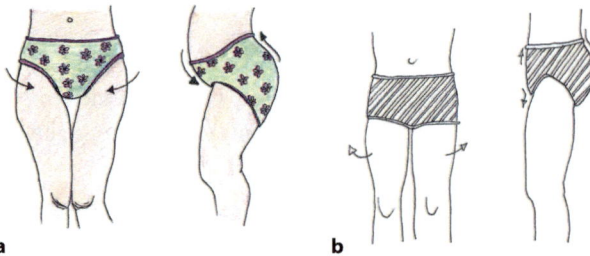

a b

◘ Fig. 9.7 a Tipped pelvis (Waldhör). b Erect pelvis (Waldhör)

9.4.2   The Axes of the Legs

The axes of the legs should be as straight as possible between the two poles – feet and pelvis. When a child stands the inner sides of the knees and ankles should just touch, then the legs are parallel and symmetric and the patellae point directly forwards. If only the knees or only the ankles touch each other, then the child has either knock-knees or bow-legs (see Fig. 9.8a,b). It can also be that only the lower legs are not straight; that is called tibia vara.

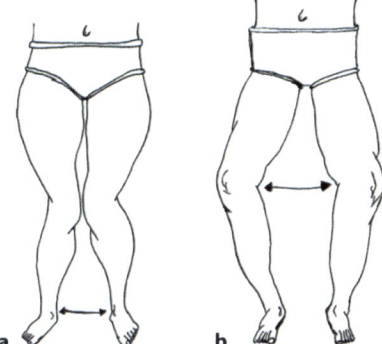

a   b

▣ Fig. 9.8 a Knock-knees (Waldhör). b Bow-legs (Waldhör)

9.5   The Development of the Foot and the Axes of the Legs During Growth

9.5.1   The Newborn

Newborns very often have a harmless deformity of the feet, such as pes adductus (pes metatarsus varus) or pes calcaneus (talipes calcaneus). The feet were pressed tightly in the confined space of the uterus; this grows out quite naturally in the first month. Sometimes an unnatural shape remains; this can be improved or corrected during childhood.

A baby trains the development of the arches by bringing the foot, especially the big toe, to the mouth. The flexion of the hip joints in abduction and external rotation, the flexion of the knee and the supination of the foot foster the development of the three-dimensional arched structure of the foot (cf. Zukunft-Huber et al. 2011).

9.5.2   The Infant

The foot bones of the infant are still soft cartilage and without the recognisable arches. This congenital flatfoot changes once the infant begins to bear weight. The foot develops from the inside once the muscles are activated by weight bearing, and during the process of learning to walk the arches take shape. Children experiment with different ways of standing, e. g. on tiptoe, until their sensory perception enables them to find a stable position (cf. Köhler,

Reber 2006). For the development of a varied motor function of the foot it is important to walk with bare feet as much as possible. In the infant the tibia forms a plateau, which means that the knee cannot be completely extended. This gives the impression of bow-legs, which like the flatfoot disappear during growth.

9.5.3 The Toddler

In toddlers bow-legs or knock-knees are connected to the state of growth of the legs and are normal. They change from one to the other and show the complexity of growth dynamics (see Fig. 9.9).

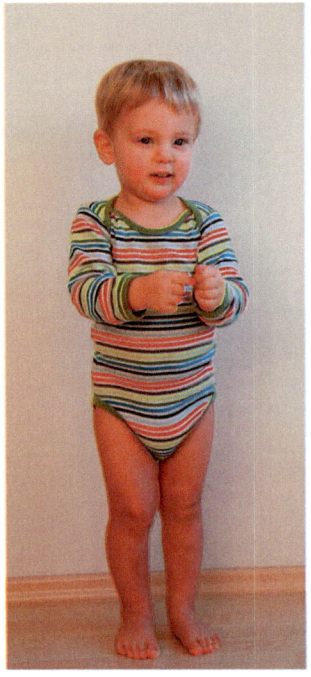

◘ **Fig. 9.9** Feet and leg axes in toddlers

By the time of transition from toddler to child, about the same time as the milk teeth begin to loosen, the leg and foot positions should have normalised: the feet should be parallel and the patellae facing forward when standing.

There are, however, many children who continue to have these leg positions after this age and do not stand straight. When standing on tiptoe the pull of the lower leg muscles should put this right (cf. Kempf, Fischer 2004).

9.5.4 The Schoolchild

Ideally, schoolchildren should have straight legs and the arches of the feet should be fully developed (see Fig. 9.10).

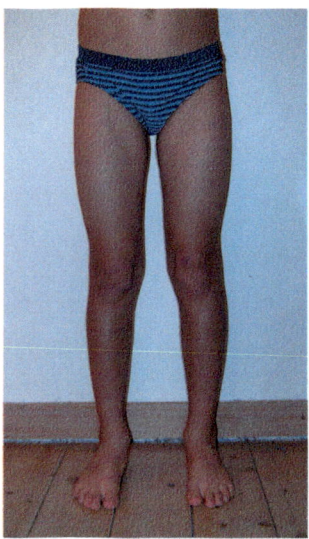

■ **Fig. 9.10** Feet and leg axes of an 8-year-old child

Unfortunately, this is frequently not the case. Poor shoes and too little weight bearing with low demands of motor adaptation leave the feet underdeveloped. The most common malpositions are pes planovalgus or talipes cavovalgus.

9.5.5 Considerations Relating to the Foot Positions and Leg Axes in People with EB

(See Fig. 9.11.a,b)
The way the positioning of the feet and the axes of the legs develop will depend on the EB type and sub-type, and the corresponding weight-bearing abilities of the feet. This may result in anything from a typical physiological position to a severe malposition.

Sensorimotor perception is reduced by the constant bandaging of the feet when a toddler with EB learns to walk.

Incorrect leg axes and position of the pelvis are the results of relieving postures of the lower extremities because of the limited weight-bearing capacity.

In severe cases of EB the feet are placed only very carefully on the ground, depending on the condition of the skin. In this way no active erect alignment of the pelvis develops and it remains tipped forwards. The knees have a tendency to knock, the thighs are rotated inwards and the foot arches are flattened. There is an apparent knock-knees position of the legs.

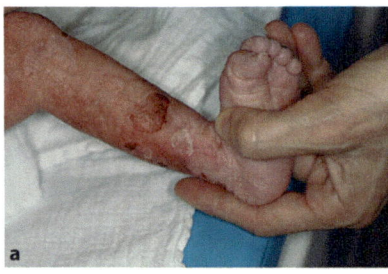
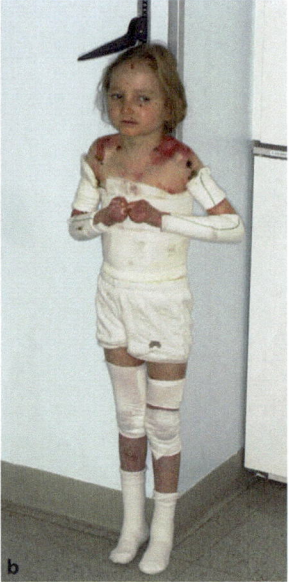

Fig. 9.11 a Foot of an infant with EB (Hametner). **b** Feet and leg axes of a schoolchild with EB (Hametner)

9.6 Malpositions of the Foot

9.6.1 Pes (Talipes) Valgus/Varus

The pes or talipes valgus is the most common and severe malposition in children. The classical type is turned inwards. Looked at from the back there is a curved axis from the heel towards the calf. The talipes valgus can be on one or both feet. The heel takes the weight incorrectly, and so forces bring about a distortion of the arches; in time they become flattened.

The second type, pes or talipes varus, shows a tipping of the calcaneus in the opposite direction (see Fig. 9.12b).

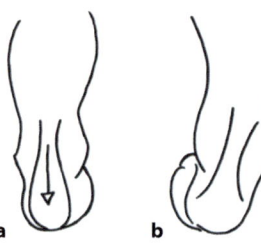

Fig. 9.12 a Foot in an upright position (Waldhör). **b** Talipes varus (Waldhör)

9.6.2 Fallen Arches, Pes Planus (Flatfoot), Pes Planovalgus

The footprint when standing is a good indication of the functional height of the arch. In a normal case, the narrowest place, the isthmus, is one third of the forefoot. In the case of fallen arches, it is two thirds of the width of the forefoot, and with flatfoot the isthmus is as wide as the forefoot. When the mid-foot is even wider than the forefoot, it is called pes planovalgus.

In the pes planovalgus the arch has no torsion, the screw principle of the bones is weakened, the cuneiform bones become unstable, and the arches are completely flattened and nullified.

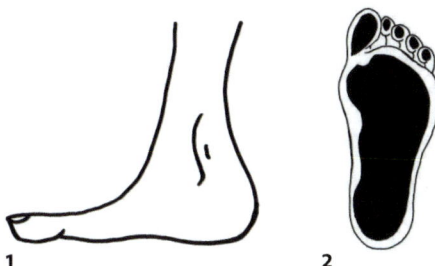

◘ Fig. 9.13 Fallen arches (Waldhör)

9.6.3 Pes Excavatus (High-Arched Foot)

Pes excavatus presents a rigid immobile mid-foot with a high instep. The spiralling is exaggerated and too strong, presenting the opposite effect of a weakened spiral function as in flatfoot (see Chap. 9.6.2). Mostly, the toes take on a claw position.

There is also a form of the pes excavatus where the calcaneus tips medially; this is a combination of the pes valgus and the pes excavatus in which the foot muscles (quadratus plantae, abductor hallucis, abductor digiti minimi, and flexor digitorum brevis) have an extremely high tone.

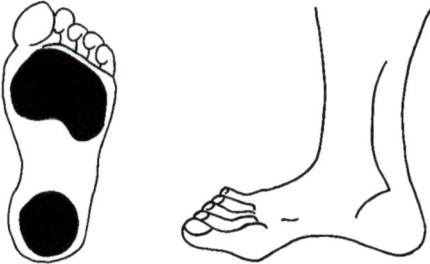

◘ Fig. 9.14 Pes excavatus (Waldhör)

The footprint of a high-arched foot is divided in two with a print of the balls of the toes and the heel; when standing, a pencil can be pushed through between these two contact points.

9.6.4   Pes Transversoplanus (Splayfoot)

The pes transversoplanus is a result of a flattening of the transverse arch. There is no or little tonicity and elasticity of the muscles and tendons. The forefoot appears flat and the foot is unproportionately wide for its length.

The flattening of the transverse arch results in the toes being overextended and not lying flat on the ground. In time claw toes develop. In extreme cases there can be a subluxation of the MTP joints. The strain on the balls of the feet often results in the development of callus.

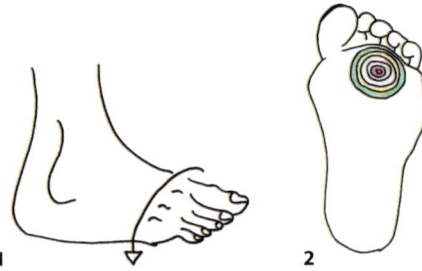

◘ Fig. 9.15 Pes transversoplanus (Waldhör)

9.6.5   Considerations Relating to the Foot in People with DEB

The condition of the skin and the adhesions of the toes correlate with the type of malposition that develops over the years (see Fig. 9.16a–d).

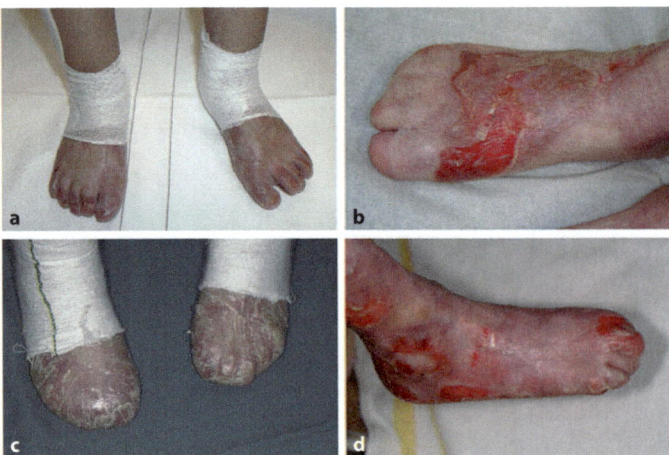

◘ Fig. 9.16 a Feet with isolated toes. **b** Adhesions of the toes without the big toe (Hametner). **c** Feet with adhesions of the toes (Hametner). **d** Severe toe deformities (Hametner)

The webbing on the toes, which is not normally removed by surgery, leads to major restrictions of movement and function of the toes. This results in the inability during locomotion to push the foot off from the ground satisfactorily in each step, and leads on to the atrophy of the small muscles and changes in the coordination of balance in the feet.

It could also be observed that webbing influences growth: if the severity of the webbing of the two feet is different, the more severely affected foot grows longitudinally (in the length) distinctly slower and remains shorter (see Fig. 9.17).

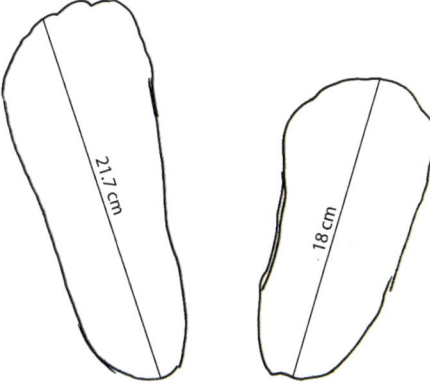

21.7 cm

18 cm

🔲 **Fig. 9.17** Feet of a 13-year-old boy. Left foot without webbing, right foot distinct webbing. Size difference of 3.7 cm

9.7 Assessment

A picture of the foot can be made for assessment purposes. A colour footprint is the most effective. If this is not possible for someone with EB, then drawing around the foot while weight bearing is the next alternative. Attention must be paid to draw only around those parts of the foot which are in contact with the ground. Great care is needed around the longitudinal arch.

This footprint shows the relationship between the width of the mid-foot, the isthmus and the width of the forefoot, which makes it possible to define the malposition of the foot.

Measuring the Transverse Arch – Pes Transversoplanus
When standing the distance between the first and second metatarsal is measured; it should be between 5 and 10° (see Fig. 9.18).

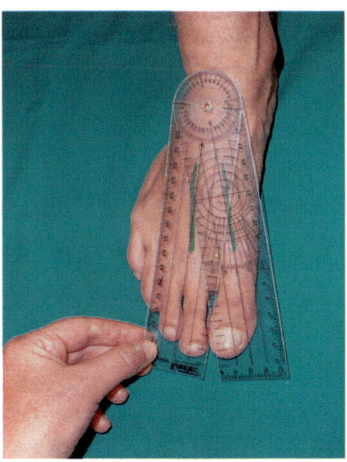

🔲 **Fig. 9.18** Assessment of pes transversoplanus (splayfoot)

Measurement of the Angle of the Heel – Pes Valgus/Varus

When standing the angle on the heel between the axis of calcaneus and the axis of the lower leg is measured. A pes valgus is present when the angle is more than 10° towards the midline, a pes varus when it is greater than 0° laterally (see Fig. 9.19).

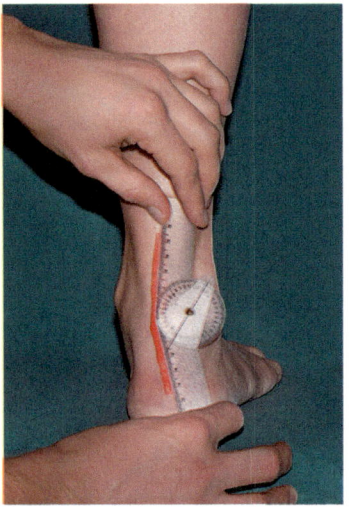

◘ **Fig. 9.19** Measuring the pes valgus (Matschi)

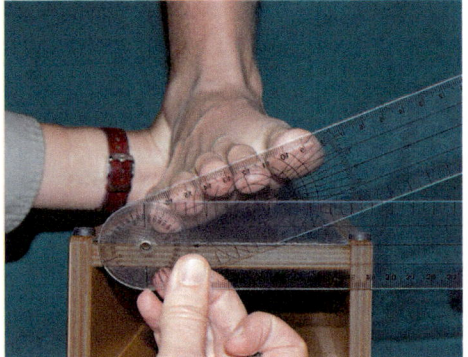

◘ **Fig. 9.20** Measuring inversion and eversion (Matschi)

Measuring Pro- and Supination (Inversion and Eversion)

The starting position is sitting with the lower leg vertical and an angle of 90° between the talocrural (ankle) joint and the orthograde heel. The inversion varies between 15 and 30°, the eversion between 30 and 60°. The relationship between pro- and supination is about 1:2 (see Fig. 9.20).

Measuring the Extension of the Talocrural (Ankle) Joint

The starting position should be squatting, but with the knees in extension (standing) the value should be the same. Dorsal extension is normally 20–30° (see Fig. 9.21).

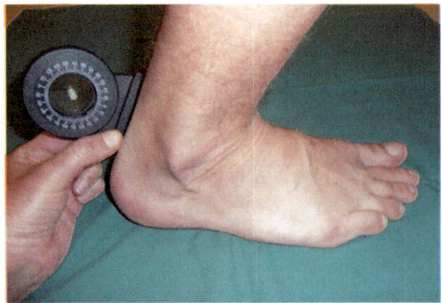

◘ **Fig. 9.21** Measuring the talocrural joint (Matschi)

ASSESSMENT FORM – FOOT

Patient:	Date of birth:
Date:	Tel.:
Diagnosis:	
School/profession:	Therapist:
	Doctor:
Special notes:	
Aims of intervention:	

Left	INSPECTION	Right
☐	State of the tissue (colour, trophic changes)	☐
☐	Blisters (where?)	☐
☐	Scars (where?)	☐
☐	Hyperkeratosis	☐
☐	Muscle atrophy (where?)	☐
	Foot deformities	
☐	Pes valgus/varus	☐
☐	Fallen arches	☐
☐	Pes planus (flatfoot)	☐
☐	Pes planovalgus	☐
☐	Pes excavatus (high-arched foot)	☐
☐	Pes transversoplanus (splayfoot)	☐
	Leg axes	
☐	Bow-legs	☐
☐	Knock-knees	☐
☐	Tibia vara	☐

Left	Footprint – Width of isthmus	Right
☐	Isthmus 1/3 of forefoot width – normal	☐
☐	Isthmus 2/3 of forefoot width – fallen arches	☐
☐	Isthmus equals forefoot width – pes planus (flatfoot)	☐
☐	Isthmus wider than the forefoot – pes planovalgus	☐
☐	Isthmus less than 1/3 or not present – pes excavatus (high-arched foot)	☐
	RANGE OF MOTION (ROM)	
	Supination/pronation ROM <45°	
☐	Contracted pes valgus/varus	☐
☐	Contracted pes planovalgus	☐
☐	Rigid pes excavatus	☐
	Supination/pronation ROM >45°	
☐	Flexible pes planovalgus	☐
☐	Flexible pes excavatus	☐
	Talocrural joint ROM <30°	
☐	Insufficient	☐
	Talocrural joint ROM >30°	
☐	Sufficient	☐
	PAIN	
☐	Where exactly?	☐
	What does it feel like?	
	When?	
☐	At rest	☐
☐	Movement	☐
☐	Weight bearing	☐
☐	Pressure pain (where?)	☐
	ACTIVE CORRECTION OF THE DEFORMITIES	
☐	Possible	☐
☐	Impossible	☐

9.8 Exercises

9.8.1 Exercises for the Perception of the Feet

The contact senses such as touch, balance and movement are important to a toddler for the orientation in the environment. From the fifth year, the distal senses such as seeing and hearing become more important. In training perception, attention should be given to one part of the body so that it can be discriminated from other parts. This discrimination can be described and brought into relation to other perceptions. Through this, the equilibrium of the body and muscle tone can be experienced and learnt (cf. Kempf, Fischer 2004).

The improved perception of foot and leg position can have a long-term effect on posture and increase the flexibility to adjust adequately to new situations.

Footprint

The child can make footprints and handprints by drawing the outlines on a piece of paper and then colouring them (see Fig. 9.22). On the foot, the areas where the floor is felt most can then be especially marked.

Another suggestion is to draw the areas where the weight should be taken into an outline of the foot. The therapist can give some help by standing the child on the outline and touching the heel and balls of the foot to draw attention to the main areas that take the weight in standing and to possibly raise an awareness of the arches. The child could have the outline in his/her room and stand on it a few times during the day to train and to practise how it should be putting his/her weight on his/her feet. Furthermore, the child needs to learn how to place the feet parallel to each other.

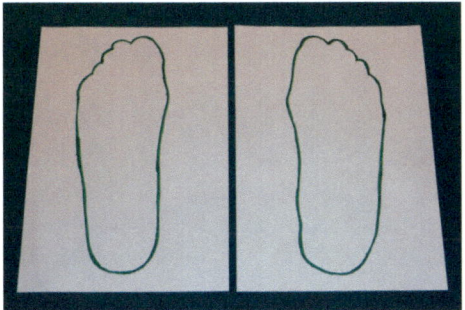

◘ Fig. 9.22 Outlines of parallel feet

Foot Training Course

Household objects such as a sponge, a wooden spoon, plastic containers, fur, brushes, rounded stones, etc. are placed on the floor. These objects should not of course present any danger of injury (see Fig. 9.23).

The child with EB can tread on these objects and feel and be aware of the feel of them, even with bandages on the feet. Then the child can be helped through the training course to feel and describe them without looking – blindfolded.

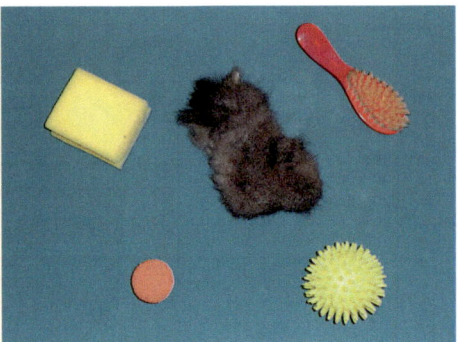

Fig. 9.23 Foot training course with different objects

'Walking' on the Wall

The child lies on his/her back close to the wall so that the hips and knees are at a right angle and the feet are against the wall. In this position the child discovers the variety of movements the feet can make: first the complete sole of the foot is placed on the wall, then the outer and the inner edges, and finally the toes, the balls of the feet and the heels. The feet can be moved in the same rolling motion from heel to toe as in walking, or from the toe to the heel. Then the feet can be positioned higher or lower so that the ankle joint becomes more bent or stretched. Ab- and adduction of the legs can provide greater pressure on the outer or inner edges of the feet and thereby also mobilise the talocrural (ankle) joint (see Fig. 9.24).

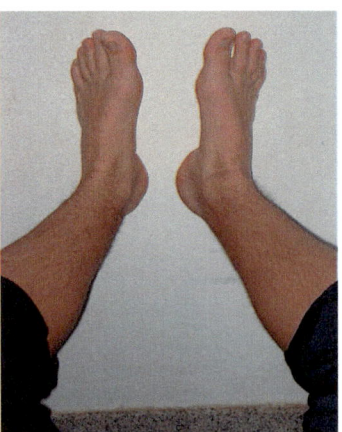

Fig. 9.24 'Walking' on the wall

Balance Bubble

The child can place the foot on a balance bubble and move it in different directions to feel where there is pressure and where the air is pushed away (see Fig. 9.25).

The perceptual exercise can move smoothly into a physical exercise by then also training the spiral movement of the foot.

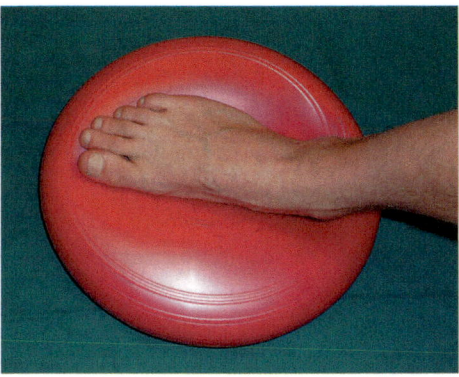

■ **Fig. 9.25** Exercise for perception with a balance bubble

Tactile Perception

The soles of the child's feet, with or without bandages, are stimulated with different materials such as brushes, fur, rough or smooth objects, rounded or cornered shapes, etc. (see Fig. 9.26). The choice of materials must be suitable for the child and situation. This exercise can be done with open or closed eyes.

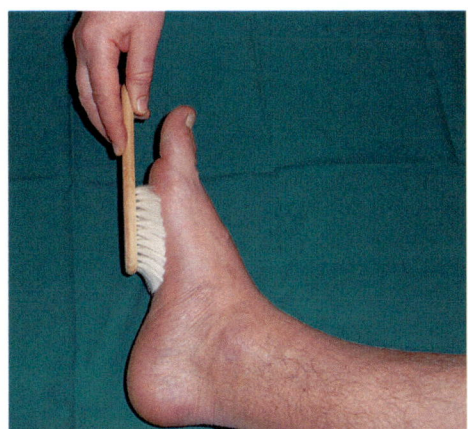

■ **Fig. 9.26** Tactile perception

Foot Massage

It is best to be sitting on the floor; massage the sensitive skin of the foot with great care. The muscles of the foot can be gently kneaded and the arches of the foot either formed or just followed through.

In this way, the perception of the feet is improved. Everything that the child can appreciate is allowed. The feet have to carry a big load so they should also be given attention and 'spoilt'. People with EB love a massage, as far as it is possible. It can also be carried out during the personal hygiene routines.

9.8.2 General Functional Exercises

'Tree in the Wind'

The child stands with the feet parallel to each other and weight bearing, as far as the state of the skin allows, correctly. Then the child should imagine that a strong wind is blowing from different directions and his/her body should sway like a tree in the wind. The feet must remain firmly in contact with the ground. Someone can also pat balloons to the child, who should catch them without moving the feet. This exercise requires a great deal of skill in keeping balance and stabilising the whole body.

Variation: Different surfaces can be used to stand on, e. g. sand outside, a foam rubber mat or padding which provide an unstable base. In this way the demands on the proprioception are increased and there is greater activity of the stabilising muscle groups. Thus, the differentiated motor adaptations that have to be made by the foot muscles can gradually be increased. The child becomes accustomed to adjusting to different kinds of ground surfaces (see Fig. 9.27).

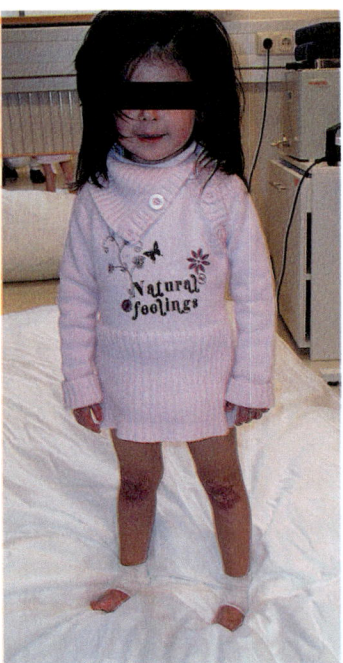

Fig. 9.27 'Tree in the wind' – coordination of the feet

Foot Theatre

The foot theatre diverts attention to the feet and allows for a variety of movements. It can be done just as well singly as in groups. The child sits on the ground and the body is covered. The feet must move in different directions and the toes begin to 'speak' to another. The foot theatre can be combined with sayings, music or stories. Faces can be drawn on the feet (see Fig. 9.28).

A single child can be placed in front of a mirror and the drawn face can take on different shapes or roles.

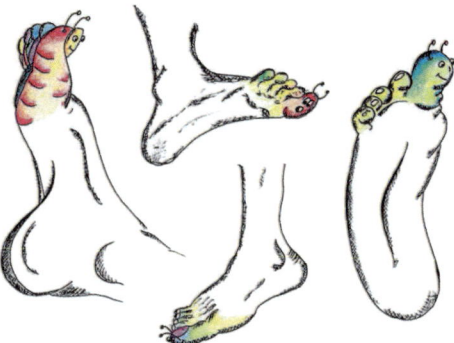

● Fig. 9.28 Foot theatre – different movements (Waldhör)

Balancing Board

With DEB children it is advisable to do these exercises in sitting. The child should place his/her feet on the board and take care to keep them on the board while it moves. There are some boards which allow movement only in two planes, e.g. flexion and extension or in- and eversion. With other models movement is possible in all directions from one swivel. The board can also be rolled along the outer edge in a circle. In this way, the child can train the muscle adjustment in a variety of directions by keeping his/her feet steadily on the board (see Fig. 9.29).

One way to make the balancing board attractive to older children is to make a shallow shape in the board (e.g. a circle, square or a figure 8, etc.), place a marble in the form and, by the movement of the board, allow the marble to run around the shape.

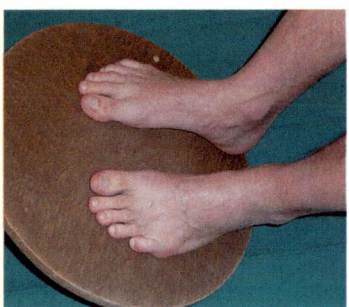

● Fig. 9.29 Balancing board

9.8.3 Mobilisation

Transverse Arch – Pes Transversoplanus (Splayfoot)

The impulse for keeping an upright posture of the whole body stems from the transverse arch. A flat arch can be mobilised by stabilising the joints on the sides of the foot and raising the middle joints – the thumbs are placed over the MTP joints of the big and little toes while the fingers lie across the balls of the foot. The arch is formed, then let go, and the foot is relaxed without compression or crushing (see Fig. 9.30).

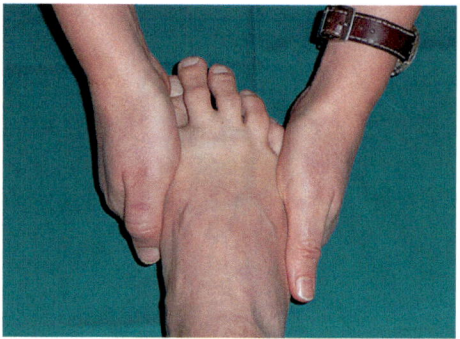

Fig. 9.30 Mobilising the transverse arch

The Longitudinal Arch or Foot Spiral – Fallen Arches and Flatfoot

The child sits on the floor and the therapist sits beside his/her feet facing away from the child. The ankle is kept at a right angle, the heel is in the therapist's hand, and the other hand holds the ball of the foot and the big toe from below. The back of the foot is moved in the direction of eversion (supination) and the forefoot in inversion (pronation) at the same time so that a spiral motion occurs. Then the foot is allowed to relax but not moved in the opposite direction before the spiralling motion is repeated. The mobilisation and relaxation should be a dynamic, fluid movement (see Fig. 9.31).

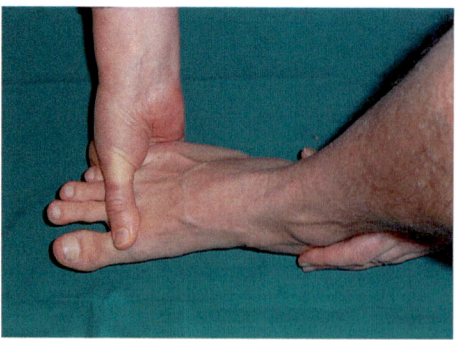

Fig. 9.31 Mobilising the foot spiral

Another mobilisation method is the neurophysiological, three-dimensional manual foot therapy. This soft tissue technique is carried out in a three-dimensional pattern of movement from the hip joints to the foot so as to prevent the carryover of malpositions from one joint to the next. Contractures in the complete chain are reduced or eliminated and the joint positions normalised (cf. Zukunft-Huber et al. 2011).

The Longitudinal Arch or Foot Spiral – Pes Excavatus (High-Arched Foot) and Claw Toes

The mobilisation is performed similarly to that of the fallen arches and flatfoot but in the opposite direction: There should be an 'unscrewing' of the foot and a lengthening of the longitudinal arch. The muscles of the sole of the foot should be relaxed and any hypertonus reduced.

The mobilisation of the joints and muscles should give the foot a better contact with the floor.

9.8.4   Functional Exercises for the Malpositions of the Foot

Pes Valgus/Varus
Sunrise/Sunset

On a sock or bandage draw the vertical axis on the heel and a sun on the inside of the foot, in the area of the tarsal bones and just below the ankle bone. The aim of the exercise is to correct the pes valgus/varus and to stretch the longitudinal arch correctly. The child tries to allow the sun to rise by raising the mid-foot and to set by lowering the mid-foot so that the longitudinal arch is stretched and the pes valgus/varus reduced. It should be noted that the foot becomes somewhat shorter because of the arching; the toes should remain relaxed.

Fallen Arches and Flatfoot
Drawing with the Feet

The foot spiral is exercised by using cream or shaving foam to draw on a mirror. The cream or foam is put onto the tip of the big toe and the child directed to 'draw' on the mirror with it.

If there are no adhesions of the toes, the foot muscles can be activated by drawing on paper, with a pen held between the first and second toe. The pen should be held so that the intrinsic muscles are active but the toes are not drawn into a claw position (see Fig. 9.32).

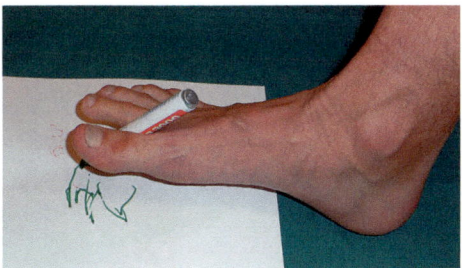

◘ Fig. 9.32 Drawing with the foot

Foam Machine

This exercise is performed when bathing. Most children prefer bathing to showering because the water-soaked dressings are easier to remove.

Sitting in the bath the child pumps a sponge with the feet; the MTP joint of the big toe mainly exerts pressure. With pressure and release in quick succession a 'cloud of foam' is formed.

Foot Pendulum

The starting position is lying on the back with knees bent and the feet placed flat on the surface a little apart, about the width of the hips. At the beginning, the heels should be vertical and the mid-foot spiralled with the weight on the MTP joint of the big toe. The therapist takes care that the position is correct. Then the child allows the knees to fall outwards as far as possible while retaining contact with the base surface at the MTP I joint. The therapist provides contact at this point to ensure a better awareness of the exercise.

This position is held for 5 s and then the knees are brought together again so that they nearly touch each other. While the knees are moved outwards, the forefoot should be actively inverted, and when the knees are brought together again there should be eversion in the back of the foot (see Fig. 9.33).

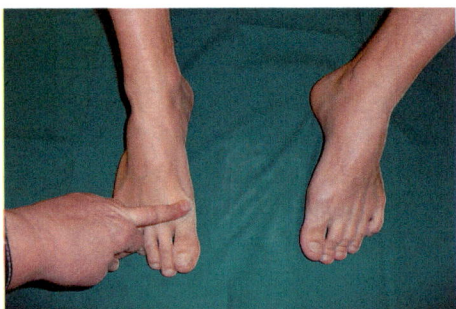

🔘 **Fig. 9.33** Foot pendulum – big toes remain on the base surface

Foot Cave

This exercise is done for talipes valgus, fallen arches and flatfoot – when there is no visible instep. The task is to make a cave on the inside of the foot; this cave can serve as a home for animals or a garage for small cars (see Fig. 9.34).

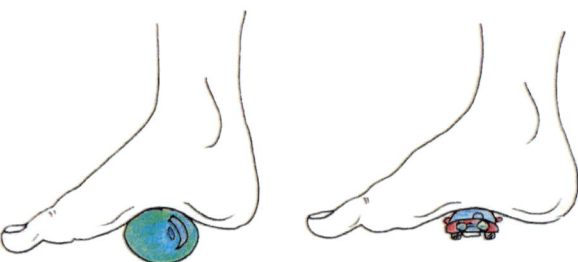

🔘 **Fig. 9.34** Foot cave – building the longitudinal arch (Waldhör)

Walking in Slow Motion

Walking in slow motion should be performed step for step very slowly and with concentration on the movements. The heel is put down straight with a tensed longitudinal arch; the knee should be pointing forwards. The forefoot gives the impulse for the lift-off and after lifting the foot the toes are relaxed (see Fig. 9.35a–c).

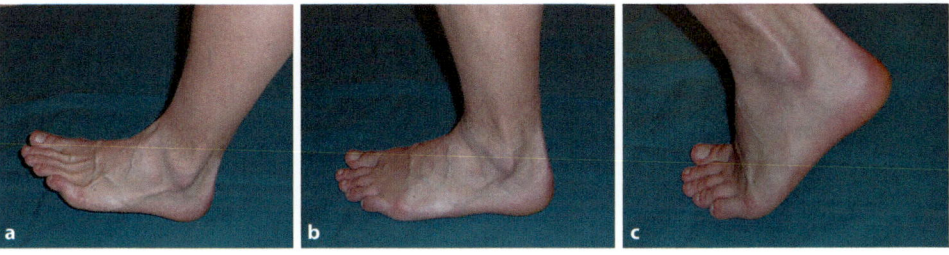

◘ Fig. 9.35 **a** Heel down with a frontal axis. **b** Foot contact with floor and spiralling. **c** Impetus for the lift-off

Pes excavatus (high-arched foot)

Contact with the floor

The patient should alternate between inversion and eversion (pro- and supination); the lack of mobility of the forefoot can be counteracted by this training. At the same time, a flattening of the longitudinal arch is aimed for by relaxing the small muscles of the mid-foot. In this way, the contact with the floor in the mid-foot region is increased.

The therapist can support the foot while the patient is learning this movement.

Pes Transversoplanus (Splayfoot)

Foot Faces

This exercise activates the muscles of the transverse arch. The eyes of a face are drawn on the skin or a sock in the areas of the MTP joints of the big and little toes, with the nose and mouth just below them. The child sits on the floor opposite a mirror. Now he/she should try to frown or wrinkle (turn up) 'the nose'. The toes should remain relaxed as far as possible.

The exercise can be given support by putting a little pressure on 'the nose' so that there is an impulse given to form the transverse arch. On the dorsal side of the foot a flat, tensed C-arch should be visible (see Fig. 9.36).

The exercise is quite difficult and it requires endurance; it is therefore more suitable for older children who already know other foot exercises.

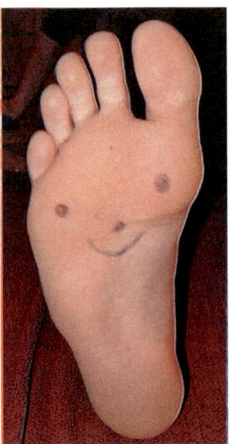

◙ **Fig. 9.36** Foot face

Peanut Bowl

A little bowl is formed in the ball of the foot by bringing the balls of the big and little toes together. In imagination this forms a bowl that could hold peanuts, which can then be taken out with the fingers (see Fig. 9.37).

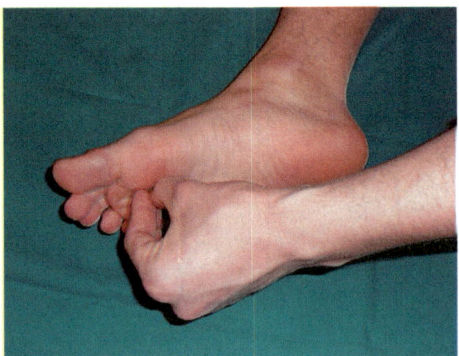

◙ **Fig. 9.37** Peanut bowl

Caterpillar Toes

For a splayfoot with fallen arches, the toes should move like little caterpillars towards the heel; with a high-arched splayfoot move in the opposite direction. The caterpillars go away from the heel pulling the foot out to be longer (see Fig. 9.38).

This exercise increases the strength of the lumbricals and interossei, and actively raises the distal transverse arch.

Caution: Exercises like ruffling up cloth or holding a pencil with the toes activate the long flexors instead of the short interossei; this can further the development of claw toes.

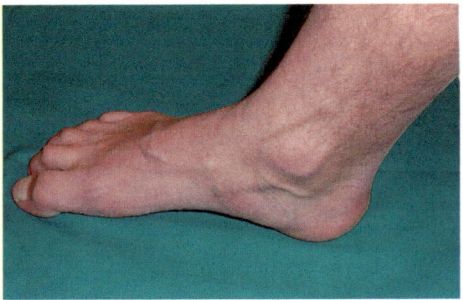

🔘 **Fig. 9.38** Caterpillar toes

Axes of the Legs

Mixing Machine

This exercise is to improve the straight axes of the legs by strengthening the outer rotation muscles, which are important for stability while walking and standing.

The child lies on the side laying his/her head relaxed on the forearm and with the underneath leg stretched. The upper leg is so placed that the foot is flat on the supporting surface. The knee is brought down to the supporting surface and then back up again as far as possible. This is repeated as often as necessary, and the 'mixing' should be as strenuous as possible. When the knee is lowered, the foot may be lifted slightly and when raising the forefoot should twist (see Fig. 9.39a,b).

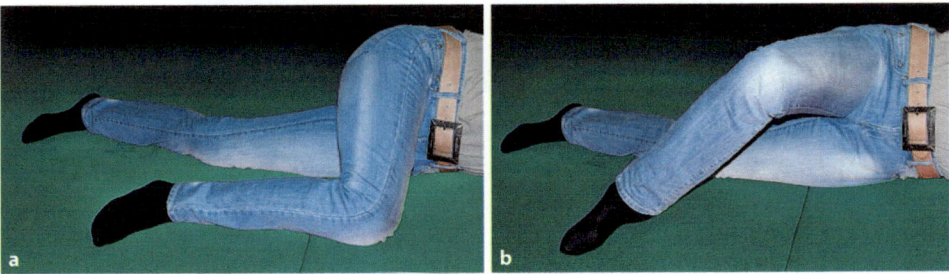

🔘 **Fig. 9.39 a** 'Mixing machine' (Matschi). **b** Activating the outer rotation muscles (Matschi)

9.8.5 Bandaging

The feet can be bandaged like the hands to prevent adhesions of the areas between the toes. The steps of bandaging are shown below (see Fig. 9.40a–f).

BANDAGING THE TOES

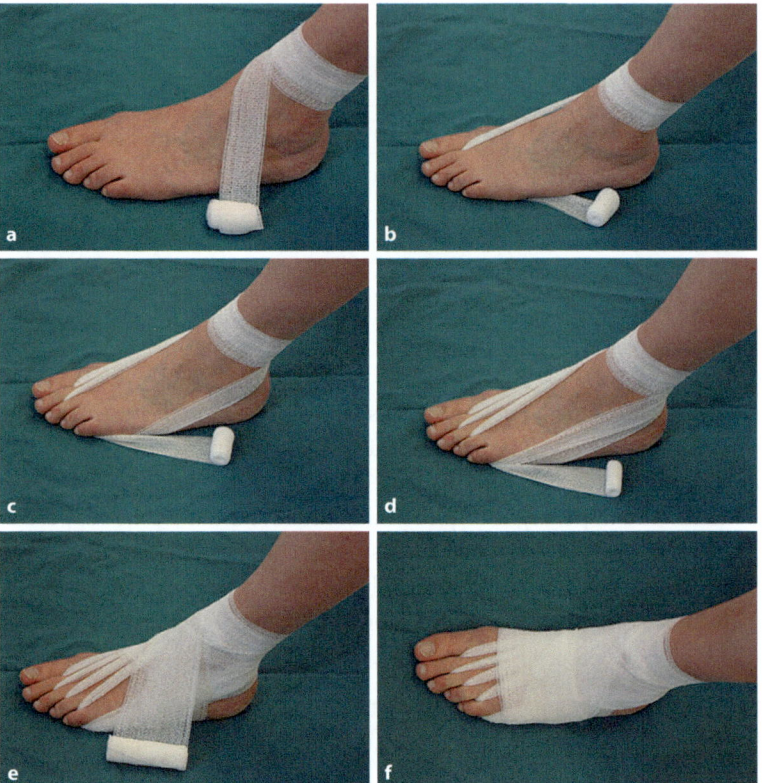

🔲 **Fig. 9.40a–f** Steps of bandaging the toes

10 Conclusion

Hedwig Weiß and Florian Prinz

The idea of this book arose out of necessity. So far, there has been no publication of OT intervention with children and youths with EB, probably because this condition is a so-called rare disease, and only a relatively small number of therapists are involved in such treatment. In therapeutic practice this meant starting with the OT treatment of EB clients on the principle of 'trial and error' or 'try and discard'. Only gradually have meaningful, goal-orientated measures with relevance to everyday life crystallised; the special needs of those affected by EB and the resulting requirements of treatment have become more distinct and clear.

A combination of paediatric OT principles and hand rehabilitation seems to offer the necessary background. Practical experience has shown that this rather unusual combination is expedient and to the point in the treatment of EB because of the very special and complex pathology. It became clear that by using a holistic approach including the entire situation of the affected person and involving OT specialists from both hand therapy and paediatrics, a much larger contribution could be made to enable EB clients their own self-determination and participation in everyday life.

In the area of motor development it can be said that the majority of children with EB show a delay of varying degrees in their early motor development. Blistering and pain cause significant problems for the child holding a prone position, thus leading to difficulties with creeping and crawling. Many children sit passively for a long time and avoid changing position. This then often delays the beginning of standing and walking. Early OT intervention in the motor development, especially in the case of DEB and – depending on the degree of severity – in cases of EBS or JEB, is considered beneficial. Additionally, parental counselling about how to encourage the motor skills at home has proved to be meaningful and supportive. Both in therapy and in the support at home a healthy balance between avoiding increased blistering and causing sores and encouraging the natural behaviour patterns of movement must be found.

Considering the factors restricting the early motor development in EB, it may be assumed that the frequently observed deficits in the vestibular and proprioceptive skills may be explained by the lack of experience. Many children move very little and very cautiously because of the limitations caused by EB. They can hardly carry out tasks that require pulling, pushing, friction or strong resistance because that would increase the blistering. Balance is also often limited by blisters on the soles of the feet and they have to take special care not to fall.

It is therefore reasonable to include the perceptual and motor development in the treatment of children with EB, which in the past has been largely neglected. The particular challenge in the intervention is to avoid pressure, friction and falls, and at the same time to give the child the opportunity of having vital vestibular and proprioceptive experiences.

Regarding the development of grip functions and dexterity, there are very different results to be observed according to the particular sub-type of the condition. As long as there are no restrictions of the fingers due to contractures, mutilations or webbing, many children show considerable dexterity in fine motor tasks. In those with DEB, in addition to the poor flexion and extension of the fingers, the mobility of the thumb is very limited: abduction and opposition often present big problems. The work pace of fine motor tasks is also often slow. However, these children are usually able to achieve a number of fine motor tasks because they compensate with bimanual grasp and with skilful use of the lateral grip, which is often possible for a long time. Therapy focuses on maintaining function for as long as possible and on learning compensation techniques and the best use of assistive devices to cope with everyday jobs.

In the area of graphomotor development, it has been shown that writing with a pen or pencil is less of a problem for children with EB than would be expected, considering the often severe deformities of the hands. In children with JEB or DEB the writing movements come more from the wrist, elbow and shoulder, thus compensating for the limited finger movement. The process of writing is thus not ergonomic and therefore more tiring. Suiting the pen to the grip abilities of the child and training the most economic compensation for the limited grip function has priority in the intervention. In cases of extreme limitation of the hand functions, the early use of a computer with any necessary adaptations of the keyboard or mouse makes sense.

Independence in everyday activities has changed quite a bit in recent years. The variety of leisure activities has increased. The possibilities of having personal assistance have improved, giving the individual greater independence. Some devices make tasks at home easier. The evaluation of the different areas of life show that coping strategies can be very different, the degree of independence of individual people with EB also varies a great deal, and the type of EB and the personality play an important role.

The results of hand rehabilitation have shown that with consistent bandaging of the interdigital spaces, the development of webbing can be delayed or even prevented. The same is true for prophylactic splinting, which can significantly affect the development of contractures of the fingers. No reliable results can be made so far regarding the use of compression gloves. The bandaging is usually well tolerated over long periods and it presents very little restriction. After years of using resting splints, they are very often rejected because the client loses the motivation, which naturally leads to a deterioration of the situation. By giving the client more choice and confining the splint to an absolute minimum (only providing the degree of correction that is absolutely necessary) and with good empathy, it is sometimes possible to bridge this period and retain the cooperation to wear the splints at least some of the time.

The results of operations with children before puberty are mostly unsatisfactory because the decision to operate is usually made by the parents. After puberty and with greater awareness of the body, youths often want to have operations on their hands. Aesthetics are usually the main reason here, because despite adhesions of the hands dexterity in everyday tasks is often good and there is no compelling necessity for an operation.

In this age group the motivation to wear splints and to carry out exercise programmes after such an operation is usually very high. Nevertheless, it must be made clear that these measures do not prevent or stop the tissue dystrophy, and so even if they are carried out with great discipline there will be no lasting result. However, it can delay the next operation quite considerably.

Feet have only recently been incorporated into the intervention. Here there are accumulated needs. The quality of gait and stamina are often seriously affected by deformities of the feet which have developed over time. To maintain long-term mobility and independence, and delay dependence on a wheelchair for as long as possible, it is important to give consideration to the feet and to posture.

In conclusion, it must be said that this book reflects the current state of therapeutic practice. Science, medicine and therapeutic approaches are all undergoing a dynamic process of development and improvement.

The authors hope that this work will provide a basis for discussion, development, change and greater quality for future OT intervention in EB.

10

Backmatter

Literature

AGR – Aktion Gesunder Rücken e.V. (2012) Ergonomic chairs and desks for children and youngsters. http://www.agr-ev.de/index.php/en/certified-and-recommended/tested-products/83-ergonomische-sitz-und-schreibmoebel-fuer-kinder-und-jugendliche. Accessed 21 Mar 2012

Ayres J (2002) Bausteine der kindlichen Entwicklung. Berlin Heidelberg New York: Springer

Becker H (2005) Kinder mit Wahrnehmungsstörungen. Idstein: Schulz-Kirchner

Becker H, Steding-Albrecht U (2006) Ergotherapie im Arbeitsfeld Pädiatrie. Stuttgart New York: Thieme

Beery KE et al (2010) Beery–Buktenica Developmental Test of Visual-Motor Integration, 6th edn (BEERY™ VMI). Pearson. http://www.pearsonassessments.com/HAIWEB/Cultures/en-us/Productdetail.htm?Pid=PAg105&Mode=summary. Accessed 26 Mar 2012

Bitzer S, Sörensen H (2010) Gelenkschutz im Alltag. Hinweise und Hilfsmittel. Bonn: Deutsche Rheuma-Liga

Brosat H, Tötemeyer N (2007) Der Mannzeichentest nach Hermann Ziler. Münster: Aschendorffsche Verlagsbuchhandlung

Burger-Rafael M (2005) Bewegungstherapie bei Schmetterlingskindern. Physikal Med Rehabilit 05/2005, p 11–12

Burger-Rafael M (2009) Physical Medicine and Epidermolysis Bullosa. In: Fine JD, Hintner H (eds) Life with Epidermolysis Bullosa (EB), Etiology, Diagnosis, Multidisciplinary Care and Therapy. Wien New York: Springer, p 278–286

Children's feet – Children's shoes (2012). http://www.kidsfeet.info. Accessed 28 Mar 2012

DEBRA International (2012) http://www.debra-international.org. Accessed 26 Mar 2012

DermaSilk (2012) http://www.dermasilk.com. Accessed 26 Mar 2012

Diem A (2009) Living with EB – Impact on Daily Life. In: Fine JD, Hintner H (eds) Life with Epidermolysis Bullosa (EB): Etiology, Diagnosis, Multidisciplinary Care and Therapy. Wien New York: Springer, p 313–333

EB Info World (2012) http://www.ebinfoworld.com. Accessed 26 Mar 2012

Eiersebner E, Prucher H (eds) (2008) Barrierefrei Bauen. Planungsgrundlagen und Praxisbeispiele. Salzburg: Land Salzburg, Abteilung Soziales

Fewtrell MS et al (2006) Bone Mineralization in Children with Epidermolysis Bullosa. Br J Dermatol; 154(5):959–962

Fine JD et al (2005) Pseudosyndactyly and Musculoskeletal Contractures in Inherited Epidermolysis Bullosa: Experience of the National Epidermolysis Bullosa Registry, 1986–2002. J Hand Surg; 30(1):14–22

Fine JD et al (2008) The Classification of Inherited Epidermolysis Bullosa (EB): Report of the Third International Consensus Meeting on Diagnosis and Classification of EB. J Am Acad Dermatol; 58:931–950

Fine JD, Mellerio JE (2009) Extracutaneous Manifestations and Complications of Inherited Epidermolysis Bullosa. Part I. Epithelial-associated Tissues. J Am Acad Dermatol; 61:367–384

Fine JD, Mellerio JE (2009) Extracutaneous Manifestations and Complications of Inherited Epidermolysis Bullosa. Part II. Other Organs. J Am Acad Dermatol; 61:387–402

Fisher AG et al (1991) Sensory Integration: Theory and Practice. Philadelphia: FA Davis Company

Greider JL, Flatt AE (1988) Surgical Restoration of the Hand in Epidermolysis Bullosa. Arch Dermatol; 124(5):765–767

Harrweg M (2006) Handrehabilitation. Wahlmodul 3 – Rheumatoide Arthritis. Fortbildung im FBA – Fortbildungsakademie für therapeutische Berufe Linz

Hochschild J (2005) Strukturen und Funktionen begreifen. Funktionelle Anatomie – Therapierelevante Details. Band 1.3.A. Stuttgart: Thieme

Jerosch-Herold C et al (2009) Konzeptionelle Modelle für die ergotherapeutische Praxis. Heidelberg: Springer

Kapandji IA (2009) Funktionelle Anatomie der Gelenke. Schematisierte und kommentierte Zeichnungen zur menschlichen Biomechanik (5). Stuttgart New York: Thieme

Keller J et al (2006) The Child Occupational Self Assessment (COSA), ver. 2.1. University of Illinois at Chicago

Kempf HD, Fischer J (2004) Rückenschule für Kinder: Haltungsschäden vorbeugen. Schwächen korrigieren. Hamburg: Rowohlt

Koesling C, Bollinger Herzka T (eds) (2008) Ergotherapie in Orthopädie, Traumatologie und Rheumatologie. Stuttgart: Thieme

Köhler B, Reber H (2006) Kinder machen Fußgymnastik. Üben mit Klein- und Schulkindern. Stuttgart New York: Thieme

Laimer M et al (2003) Epidermolysis bullosa. Pädiatrie und Pädologie; 6:30–38

Laimer M et al (2008) Epidermolysis bullosa hereditaria. Monatsschr Kinderheilkd; 156:110–121

Largo RH (2007) Babyjahre. Entwicklung und Erziehung in den ersten vier Jahren. München: Piper

Larsen C (2006) Füße in guten Händen. Spiraldynamik – programmierte Therapie für konkrete Resultate. Stuttgart: Thieme

Larsen C (2007) Gut zu Fuß ein Leben lang. Fehlbelastungen erkennen und beheben. Stuttgart: Trias in MVS Medizinverlage

Larsen C, Miescher B, Wickihalter G (2007) Gesunde Füße für Ihr Kind. Stuttgart: Trias in MVS Medizinverlage

Lauper R (2009) Von Kopf bis Fuß in Bewegung. Spielerische Körperarbeit mit Schulkindern. Zürich: Orell Füssli

Ludwikowski B (2009) Surgical Interventions. In: Fine JD, Hintner H (eds) Life with Epidermolysis Bullosa (EB), Etiology, Diagnosis, Multidisciplinary Care and Therapy. Wien New York: Springer, p 246–257

Marr D et al (2001) Handwriting Readiness: Locatives and Visuo-motor Skills in the Kindergarten Year. Early Childhood Research and Practice (ECRP), vol 3(1). http://ecrp.uiuc.edu/v3n1/marr.html. Accessed 18 Sept 2011

Mink AJF et al (2001) Manuelle Therapie der Extremitäten. Funktionsuntersuchungen und manualmedizinische Behandlungstechniken. Stuttgart: Urban and Fischer

Mullett F (1998) A Review of the Management of the Hand in Dystrophic Epidermolysis Bullosa. J Hand Ther; 11(4):261–265

Nacke A (2005) Ergotherapie bei Kindern mit Wahrnehmungsstörungen. Stuttgart: Thieme

Netzwerk EB (2009) http://www.netzwerk-eb.de. Accessed 19 Mar 2009

Pätzold I et al (2008) Weißt du eigentlich was mir wichtig ist? COSA Child Occupational Self Assessment. Dortmund: Verlag Modernes Lernen

Pikler E, Tardos A (2001) Lasst mir Zeit. Die selbständige Bewegungsentwicklung des Kindes bis zum freien Gehen. München: Pflaum

Pölzleitner MC (2007) Ergotherapie bei Epidermolysis bullosa in der Handrehabilitation. Salzburg: Akademie für Ergotherapie

Pschyrembel W (2012) Pschyrembel – Klinisches Wörterbuch (263). Berlin New York: de Gruyter

Putz T (1999) Physiotherapeutische Anwendungsmöglichkeiten bei Epidermolysis Bullosa. Unpublished diploma thesis. Wien: Akademie für den physiotherapeutischen Dienst

Rudolf H (1986) Graphomotorische Testbatterie – Manual. Weinheim: Beltz

Spiraldynamik® (2012) www.spiraldynamik.com/konzept.htm. Accessed 21 Mar 2012

Steding-Albrecht U (2003) Das Bobath-Konzept im Alltag des Kindes. Ergotherapeutische Prinzipien und Strategien. Stuttgart: Thieme

Waldner-Nilsson B et al (2009). Handrehabilitation. Grundlagen, Erkrankungen (Bd. 1). Heidelberg: Springer Medizin Verlag

Weil M, Amundson S (1994) Relationship Between Visuomotor and Handwriting Skills of Children in Kindergarten. Am J Occupat Ther; 48(11):982–988

Windsor MM (1995) Handwriting in Boys with Attention-deficit/Hyperactivity Disorder. Unpublished doctoral dissertation, Boston University

Yan EG et al (2007) Treatment Decision-making for Patients with the Herlitz Subtype of Junctional Epidermolysis Bullosa. J Perinatol; 27:307–311

Zukunft-Huber B et al (2011) Der kleine Fuß ganz groß. Dreidimensionale manuelle Fußtherapie bei kindlichen Fußfehlstellungen. München: Urban & Fischer/Elsevier

Subject Index